From the Ashes of Experience:

Reflections on Madness, Survival and Growth

Edited by
PHIL BARKER PHD, RN, FRCN,
PETER CAMPBELL BA(HONS),
BEN DAVIDSON BA (JOINT HONS), RMN

D1198115

W

WHURR PUBLISHERS

LONDON

© 1999 Whurr Publishers
First published 1999 by
Whurr Publishers Ltd
19b Compton Terrace, London N1 2UN, England

British Library Cataloguing in Publication Data
A catalogue record for this book is available from the
British Library.

ISBN 1 86156 120 2

Printed and bound in the UK by Athenaeum Press Ltd,
Gateshead, Tyne & Wear

Contents

The Editors

Phil Barker (Northumberland, England), PhD RN FRCN is a psychiatric nurse and is Professor of Psychiatric Nursing Practice in the Department of Psychiatry, University of Newcastle, England. He has published a dozen books, 30 book chapters and over 80 academic and professional papers. He has wide-ranging research interests, but is mainly interested in human questions: what is personal meaning in mental distress, and what do people need psychiatric nurses for? Email: pjbarker@newcastle.ac.uk

Peter Campbell (London, England) is a mental health system survivor. He works as a writer and freelance trainer in the mental health field. He was a founder member of Survivors Speak Out and Survivors Poetry and has been a council member of Mental Health Media for a number of years. He has contributed numerous chapters to books on mental health nursing and other mental health issues, presented many papers to interprofessional conferences and has written articles for a range of journals and publications. With Vivien Lindow, he co-authored *Changing Practice: Mental Health Nursing and User Empowerment*. Peter lives in north-west London and has written two collections of poems. A third, *A Breath Outwards*, is in preparation.

Ben Davidson (London, England) a psychiatric nurse and group analyst, is Senior Lecturer, Mental Health Nursing at South Bank University. He has published many articles, a few book chapters and an edited text (the latter with Phil Barker) on ethical issues in psychiatric nursing and other mental health issues. He co-ordinates the User Employment Project at South West London and St George's Hospital Mental Health NHS Trust (previously Pathfinder Mental Health Services NHS Trust) and sees patients for individual and group psychotherapy at the Maudsley Hospital. Email: Ben@bendavidson.freeserve.co.uk

Contributors

United States of America

Daniel B. Fisher MD PhD (Massachusetts, USA) is Executive Director of the National Empowerment Center, Lawrence, Massachusetts, and is community psychiatrist at the Riverside Mental Health Center, Wakefield, Massachusetts. He was a research scientist at the National Institute of Mental Health, Bethesda, Maryland. He has recovered from schizophrenia.

Judi Chamberlin (Massachusetts, USA) is arguably the major 'user-advocate' voice in the USA. She has published and lectured widely and has been on a number of academic journal editorial boards, concentrating now on her work on the editorial board of *Psychiatric Rehabilitation Journal.*

Sally Clay (Florida, USA) is a highly respected peer advocate in the American user-advocacy forum. She is consultant for the PEER Center, Ft. Lauderdale and for the Sanbourne class action lawsuit. She is a former trainer and therapist with the Windhorse programme in Northampton, Massachusetts. She helped establish three successful consumer-run organizations: the Portland Coalition in Maine, PEOPLe in New York, and Altered States of the Arts, a national coalition. Her writing is posted online at: http://ddi.digital.net/~sally/

Ed Manos (New Jersey, USA) is currently the Project Co-ordinator for the Compeet Program of the Catholic Charities, Diocese of Trenton, Mercer Behavioral Health Care Division. Previously, Ed worked as co-ordinator of the Collaborative Support Program (CSP) of New Jersey and Supportive Housing Initiative, a user-led housing, education and advocacy programme. Prior to working with the Consumer/Survivor Movement in New Jersey, Ed worked in direct service in the mental health system as an employment specialist, an outreach counsellor, a case manager, recreation counsellor and a 'peer advocate'. Before entering the field of human services, Ed worked in corporate private security, and criminal justice, for fourteen years.

Kate Millet (New York, USA) is author of *The Loony Bin Trip* and *Sexual Politics.*

United Kingdom

Annie T. Altschul (Edinburgh, Scotland) is Emeritus Professor of Nursing, University of Edinburgh. Professor Altschul has been a psychiatric nurse and a psychiatric patient. She described her experience of care and treatment for a psychotic depression over a decade ago in the book *Wounded Healers* (1985).

Liz Davies (Sussex, England) is a scientist and poet. She has worked as a teacher with emotionally disturbed children and adults. In earlier years she provided a home for emotionally disturbed adolescents. She now works full time as a post-doctoral scientist, researching in a field of biophysics related to medicine. She writes poetry, stories and plays, prints her own books, and is involved in a local healing circle. She is wary of being identified by her disclosure in this book of an episode of wrong diagnosis by psychiatrists. But the experience of disempowerment, psychological invalidation and humiliation also strengthened her sense of true values and her knowledge of an integral, inviolable self, which she welcomes the opportunity to share.

Jan Holloway (London, England) was born in London in 1957. She has worked as an occupational therapist since 1980, mostly in the mental health field. She has also managed a day centre for people with long-term mental health problems. She currently works for a London teaching hospital as a senior occupational therapist. She has used mental health services since 1991 and has had three in-patient admissions in psychotic states. She has learned a lot from this experience both personally and professionally, and has taken a lead role in establishing a user's forum in Newham, East London.

Rose Snow (Manchester, England) works developing user involvement and group advocacy for a user-run organization in the inner city. She has been involved for some years in developing local economies (Local Exchange Trading Schemes – LETS), and in efforts to set up a UK Spiritual Emergence Network, enriching and expanding current knowledge of psychosis. Rose is an experienced conference speaker and workshop facilitator. She has been a businesswoman and television stage manager (15 years), and one-time musician. Her most recent qualification is as a Common Purpose Graduate (1997). She is a poet and mother of two teenage sons.

Rachel E. Perkins (London, England) is a Clinical Psychologist, Director of the Rehabilitation and Continuing Care Services of an NHS Trust, and also Project Director of the User Employment Project at Springfield Hospital, South London.

Australia

Simon Champ (Sydney, New South Wales) has been a consumer activist since 1982. He has been involved in the development of the consumer movement in Australia, a process that has taken him from confrontation to co-operation as he has become involved in advising national government on mental health matters. Currently he sits on the Mental Health Council of Australia and is a director of Sane Australia. What he likes best is lecturing and speaking in public, changing minds and hearts about the potential of people who have experienced a mental illness. He is also an artist with an interest in spirituality.

Cathy Conroy (Goulburn, New South Wales) is the mother of three children. She had her first psychotic breakdown during her early teaching years. Eight years later, with the birth of her third child, she had a post-partum psychosis and was diagnosed as having a bi-polar disorder. Her professional qualifications have been in the area of education and music. She works independently as a mental health advocate for Southern Area NSW Mental Health. Her personal life experience of mental illness is the medium for her voice as an advocate.

Forewords

ANNIE T. ALTSCHUL AND KATE MILLET

It is always an honour to be invited to write a foreword. It is doubly so on this occasion because I truly belong to the fellowship of those whose voices the editors aim to bring to public attention, those who have experienced madness, who have survived and have grown as a result of the experience. Ten people describe their experiences in this book, ten very different people: different in age, in culture, in social and professional standing, different in the form of their madness and in the use of services provided for them.

I hope the readership of this book will be composed also of very different people. The stories told here will strike a chord with all those who are struggling to come to terms with problems of their own or who have done so in the past. They will also profoundly affect readers whose work brings them into contact with consumers of the psychiatric services and with the people whose plight they are dedicated to alleviating. Friends and families of those who are experiencing mental turmoil will find empathy with the storytellers. Those who believe that they are 'normal' and that madness has nothing at all to do with them may discover as they read on that no one is immune and that it is 'normal' to be mad.

What all the storytellers have in common is the way they emphatically explain how the experience of madness is incorporated in the whole of themselves. Their essential personal human *self* includes their madness. It is not a matter of 'coping' with an intrusion; it is part of the basis of their existence.

The editors elaborate on this theme, in the first and last chapters and in the commentary to each of the stories. They do this in a philosophical and psychological manner and in a way that critiques professional education. The issue of language has always been of great importance to me personally. Quite recently, in discussion of the film 'Shine', I said that it was about a mad pianist. One of my nursing friends was horrified that I should use such a word. I am delighted to find that its use is legitimized in this book. I have long struggled with the problem of discovering what would be left of *me* if attributes such as my madness were to be considered as possessions that I might lose. The current vocabulary used in the UK, concerned with 'detention' rather than with protection, care and treatment, and which has introduced the concept of 'sectioning' a person, helps, I think, to explain why some of the story writers felt they experienced incarceration.

I have always believed, and I shall continue to do so, that nurses, among other professionals, should encourage patients to talk and that they should listen with all their attention. The storytellers would agree, I think, that it was or would have been helpful to be listened to. However, reading this book confirms my belief that madness cannot be understood piecemeal either by the professional helper or by the person who is in the midst of a psychotic episode. A more complete picture is necessary to understand what the individual experience meant at the time and what effect it has on personal growth.

The value of this book is that it offers understanding as a result of its vibrant, retrospective account of Madness, Survival and Growth.

Annie T. Altschul, Edinburgh, 1999

★   ★   ★   ★

One of the books that shaped my generation is Marge Piercy's 1976 novel *Woman on the Edge of Time*, a dystopia whose Chicana heroine Consuelo Ramos is incarcerated in two different mental hospitals where she spends her time imagining a Utopia placed far in the future after we have all learned a better way to live. Betrayed into Bellevue by relatives and tied into four-point restraint under heavy sedation she is left for days to lie in her own urine or to choke on her own vomit or simply to die of despair.

The terror and humiliation of such capture matches anything our century has to offer in the literature of political imprisonment or torture. Yet it is not an uncommon experience in our time. Sudden arrest and incarceration in a mental hospital is recounted by a number of those who testify in this volume. Among those who participate in the international movement against psychiatric abuse there is hardly anyone who has not undergone this devastating trauma. Deprived of all civil or even human rights through 'diagnosis' under the intellectually dishonest and scientific-ally invalid mechanism of the psychiatric 'medical model', one loses all existence as a person or citizen under the legal doctrine of 'substituted judgement' and becomes a 'mental patient', a creature without hope or decision, deprived of all access to one's own money or resources and denied even liberty of person, a captive without rights or representation.

Felons are far better off. Their alleged crimes are acts separate from their essence; even convicted they remain worthy of consideration as reasonable beings, whereas those accused of 'madness' are convicted through the very accusation; the taint of unreason deprives them of every entitlement. The very term 'mental patient' and the subhuman status it implies, this unique category of nonentity, is an anomaly in modern civil life and one that cries out for scrutiny as a human rights abuse.

Seen in this light there are many human rights abuses perpetrated by psychiatry and put forth as treatments: lobotomy, electro-convulsive shock, four-point restraint, forced drugging and involuntary confinement. These activities are protected by the prestige of science and medicine but without such defence they would be regarded simply and logically as forms of torture.

Psychiatry and its practices are all supported ultimately by the use of force and police powers, legal procedure and state power. Even where supported by popular belief and social assent they are routinely performed against the wishes and interests of their victims since psychiatry depends finally and stubbornly on its state-licensed entitlement to the involuntary treatment of its designated subjects.

The power of psychiatry has grown enormously in our century – making cause with the interests of governmental control and continuously licensed and empowered by it and the network of social agencies that weave together and unite in the present Therapeutic State. This extremely effective form of social control is now proliferating around the world through the spread of dominant ideology and a carefully created popular faith in 'mental health', spreading the offices of psychiatric authority over behaviour worldwide. With this comes the economy of pharmacological profit, manufacture and maintenance. Whole populations never before exposed to either are now introduced to each as signs of modernism and progress.

Much of what psychiatry has achieved against individual freedoms is opposed by groups of 'survivors' – persons who have not only experienced psychiatric abuse but also address the climate of intellectual conformity psychiatry has created: its persecution of eccentricity and the imaginative and even the spiritual element in human thought. Taking issue with the specious logic of psychiatry's 'medical model' (that psychic dis-ease is analogous to physiological pathology) they see their mission as the defence of reason as well as imagination and the multiplicity and variety of mental experience.

The reliance upon force – indeed the refusal to relinquish the use of force – was made clear at the Foucault Tribunal in Berlin in May of 1998, when psychiatry was 'put on trial' for human rights abuse by the Irren Offensive – a group of German psychiatric survivors – in a two-day theatrical event sponsored by the Free University of Berlin and held at Bertolt Brecht's hallowed Volksbuhne Theatre. The Chief Psychiatrist of the State Mental Hospital at Bremen stalwartly represented psychiatric science before the Tribunal's charges but was candid in his refusals to forgo the use of force – including state and police force – in treatment. The outcome of the Tribunal, an exercise in debate and the drama of ideas, was sealed in this refusal: psychiatry was found guilty of human rights offences.

But as with most human rights efforts, the first thing to address is the instance of greatest suffering. The outcome of the Foucault Tribunal was predicated upon psychiatry's insistence on the use of force. But so was the determination of the participants and their fellow survivors to bring their claims to a higher court than the theatre of ideas. Observing how Amnesty International and other voluntary non-governmental organizations operating under the auspices of the United Nations have been successful on behalf of political prisoners and victims of torture, the movement against psychiatric abuse is now organizing towards recognition by the United Nations for non-governmental status. As this is achieved, it can address specific psychiatric abuses (psycho-surgery, electro-shock, restraint, forced drugging and involuntary confinement) as offences against the Universal Declaration of Human Rights.

Kate Millet, New York, 1999

Preface

A central feature of the predicament of people who 'use' mental health services is the apparent difficulty of viewing their life as a whole. Mental health professionals and other social care workers, alongside non-experts, find it easier to focus on discrete elements in the individual's life: their 'illness', their service use, their housing need. For many societies, the diagnosed-mentally-ill as *service user* or *consumer of mental health care* appears to be easier to countenance than the diagnosed-mentally-ill as citizen or human being. Thus, although mental health services increasingly acknowledge the important contribution within those services of people who 'use' or otherwise receive psychiatric care, and although the need to foster collaborative relationships with service users and their families is mandatory in the UK and other Western societies, the proposition that mental health service users have a positive contribution to make in the wider society is still controversial.

The contemporary interest in involving service users in their own care and treatment, or as advocates in the care of others, derives in part from the philosophical and political critiques of traditional psychiatry that emerged at the end of the 1960s in both the USA and Europe. Some European political initiatives based on the ideas of community development and action originating with Freire in Brazil – in particular Psichatria Democratica in Italy – demonstrated how institutional psychiatric services could be remodelled and integrated into communities, prioritizing desegregation and citizenship. Some smaller-scale, 'non-institutional' initiatives, such as the Kingsley Hall experiment in London in the late 1960s, attempted to emphasize more the core *humanity* of the people involved, while their leading exponents proselytized as to the developmental and spiritual potential of such people's experiences: breakdown as, at least potentially, break*through*.

Nevertheless, although such initiatives have often articulated the values and beliefs shared by many mental health service users, it has sometimes been ideas from a slightly different source that have ignited activity in a particular country. In the United Kingdom, for example, a major stimulus to the growth of action came from the ubiquity of health service consumerism, with its recognition of the 'mental patient' as consumer and acknowledgement of the validity of direct evidence from such consumers in planning, delivering and monitoring psychiatric services. Although this vision is not the vehicle for the dreams of Kingsley Hall, or of today's radicals, it has already carried the involvement of mental health service users a good way forwards.

The pattern of development for service user action inevitably varies from country to country. Even so, there are strong common elements. Life with a mental illness diagnosis in any Western industrialized society has many similarities. When service users from different countries meet, what is remarkable is how much they share. They usually even agree as to which drugs are the worst for negative effects. The anger of individuals at the personal damage mental health services have caused is still a strong and common motivating factor, and some activists may be united more by this feeling of a common wrong than by any precise agreement on an analysis of its causes or priorities for a solution. Although in most countries activists have overcome the criticism that they have nothing positive to offer, the sense of belonging to an oppressed group remains strong. Consciousness-raising, the process through which service users talk or engage together in creative activity such as art, theatre or poetry to explore their personal experience and seek out new understandings of their situation, has been central to action in most countries.

The service user movement in each country has a unique history. But it will face similar challenges about how best to act. One key issue in this respect will be how much to become involved with the mental health system itself. Is it possible to retain control of your own agendas if you work too closely with service providers? It is interesting to note how the UK movement started from a separatist position in the early 1980s, was drawn into collaboration through government enthusiasm for 'user involvement' and is now closely tied into the service system. The UK movement has also been comparatively slow in developing self-help and user-led alternatives. In other countries such as the USA, where total opposition to compulsion became a defining point in disability politics and action, user-led initiatives have been seen as an important way forward.

Many service user activists have separated themselves from mental health professionals, to self-organize and then return to work with professionals from a position of strength. Some (probably not as many) have also worked with people from other disadvantaged/oppressed groups. In the USA, both before and since the Americans with Disabilities Act (ADA), service users and disabled people have worked together, whereas in the United Kingdom service user activists have played only a small role in civil rights campaigning. Indeed, in the UK the Employer's Forum on Disability (the EFD – self-styled as the 'CBI[1] with focus') has complained at the inactivity of mental health service users in lobbying for a stronger Disability Discrimination Act (DDA – the UK version of the ADA). The EFD claim that the DDA only went as far as it did in recognizing and protecting the interests of those with social disabilities arising from mental illness, and the stigma associated with it, as a result of their campaigning. The fact that the Chief Executive of the EFD is from a North American background with experience in operationalizing the ADA may, ironically, indeed have had more effect on the modest legal protection afforded by the DDA than any specific action by UK service users or groups.

Whether or not mental health service users should align themselves with other disabled or disadvantaged groups, the question of when to turn from the inadequacies of your particular system of psychiatric care and control to look at your position within the community remains a critical one. The position of the diagnosed mentally ill both within psychiatric services and in society generally depends on recognition of civil and human rights, on belief in a common humanity and on acknowledgement of the positive contribution that people with such diagnoses might make. Although the mental health services in numerous countries now acknowledge that the service user's direct knowledge of being in receipt of services is legitimate and vital evidence for the planning, managing and monitoring of those services, less certain is the professional reception for new understandings based on personal experience, in particular personal experience of madness[2]. The possibility that people with a mental illness diagnosis have valuable insights in these areas seems still to be approached with some reluctance. The same is probably true when considering the contribution that service users can make as providers rather than consumers of care. Although there has been gradual movement in some countries to encourage the employment of service users in mental health services, and in some cases (such as at Pathfinder Mental Health Services NHS Trust in London and statutory services in Colorado) explicitly *because of* rather

---

[1] Confederation of British Industry.
[2] The editors and contributors each define their own terms to describe the experience of 'mental breakdown', 'breakthrough', 'madness' and 'recovery' and to confer their own meanings on that experience.

than *despite* their experience, employment, if it happens at all, is more likely to occur in posts not directly involved in the provision of care. Meanwhile, most professional organizations remain profoundly ambivalent (to say the least) about having practitioners with a mental illness diagnosis.

If the proposition that service users have a positive contribution to make receives a rather guarded reception within mental health services, even less can be claimed for the response in the world beyond such services. Here, the starting point, and to some extent the end point too, is the belief that people with a mental illness diagnosis are a burden – in other words, they make a *negative* contribution. A recent poster campaign featuring the headline: 'You don't have to be mentally ill to suffer from mental illness' sums it up nicely. Faced by such rooted attitudes, it is highly unusual for high achievers to reveal a history of mental illness or madness (except in the field of creative arts). Although large numbers of people remain fascinated by the 'madness experience', this is still addressed from narrow and unrealistic viewpoints.

It could be argued that a more sensitive *appreciation* of the total reality of the 'madness experience', an appreciation of the interior perceptions, feelings, thoughts and experience, and the exterior reactions based on them, is the single most important development that could improve the quality of life of the diagnosed mentally ill. This book aims to offer just that, presenting a number of personal experiences and providing an alternative to the received wisdom that 'mental illness' is an *affliction*, an inevitably demoralizing experience, which all 'patients' would avoid if they could. This book does not aim to challenge directly the traditional canons of psychiatric medicine and psychology. Instead it offers a uniquely human, indeed, spiritual perspective on the 'madness experience' and the process of survival and subsequent human growth.

The book comprises 12 chapters. The Introduction, written by Phil Barker, Peter Campbell and Ben Davidson, provides a historical overview of the phenomenon of mental illness, its reception and the contemporary attitude toward it and toward those experiencing it.

Chapters 2–11 feature narratives on the experience of 'madness' and the receipt of psychiatric services. These narratives are written by people who have had experience of North American, British and Australian psychiatric services. The contributors comprise four American writers (two women and two men), six British writers (all women), and two Australian writers (one woman and one man). Each narrative is complemented with a commentary by the editors, aiming to draw out common themes from each of the 'patient's' experiences, and also to identify what lessons might be learned from the narratives by mental health professionals and service planners. The political emphasis of psychiatric services in the UK, the USA and the Antipodes is on people with 'serious and enduring mental illness'. All the contributors to the book have had experience of something diagnosed as a 'psychotic' disorder – either schizophrenia or manic depression.

The narratives begin with the attempt of an American woman, Sally Clay, to distinguish between *Madness and Reality*. Sally catapults the reader into her earliest experience of nightmarish oppression in the East Coast American psychiatric institution where she was first held during the 1950s. While this account opens our discourse on the politics of psychiatric power, the second part of Sally's chapter, a reconstruction of this damaging experience 30 years on, in terms of a wholly misguided response to someone who might better have been seen as a 'wounded prophet', opens our discourse linking spiritual and psychotic experience. Spiritual emergence in the individual and spiritual ignorance in society do not mix well together, and Sally's thoughts on the implications for a system of genuine mental health care rooted in spiritual vision, and professional preparation for those working in it, finds echoes in many subsequent chapters.

We then cross the Atlantic to London in the 1990s, where Jan Holloway draws our focus in somewhat in the second piece, *The Other World*. As a senior manager and clinician in the mental health system, what are the nuts and bolts of negotiating a path through a series of increasingly intense psychotic experiences, over and back across the counter separating us and them, professional and patient? Jan may offer no grander construction than that the experience has augmented her professional practice, helped her negotiation of transience and improved her ability in general to empathize, but the poignancy of her writing leaves us moved to countenance such a simple but powerful experience of madness, survival and growth.

We move on to Australia in our third narrative, *Fire and Ice*, where Cathy Conroy swoops from her flight through a garden of magically scented and coloured flowers to embrace the reader by means of a dance of poetry and prose, polemic and prayer, despair and inspiration. Cathy recounts a number of events and periods of her life, highs and lows, but the focus is ever on the way her experiences are translated into new life and creativity, especially the transition from her role as a teacher to that of advocate. The spiritual dimension of Cathy's story is explicit as she recalls the question posed by Casteneda's Yaqui Indian sage: 'Is this a path with heart?' Perhaps recovery is not about the cessation of psychiatric symptoms (in Cathy's case, intense mood swings between mania and depression), but about the way any of us, psychotic or otherwise, may harness the human capacity for regeneration and love.

This, with a more prosaic style of delivery, is essentially what Ed Manos, another American contributor, describes in our fourth piece, *The Flight of the Phoenix*. Ed's account details, however, two parallel processes: first, his own struggle to discern ways of coping with his psychiatric symptoms (with the help of lithium, marriage and work); and, second, the rise of the 'prosumer' movement. Ed's calm may spring from long years of encounter with seasonal mood swings, battle with a psychiatric system which counselled him not to expect to have a family or a life, and struggle with a suspicion that the hereditary predisposition to psychiatric problems inherited from his mother may in turn pass on to his children. But his sobriety of style also suggests a strength of character which is borne out in Ed's preoccupation with solidarity and respect, facets of mental health care too often neglected in statutory service provision. Solidarity and respect are, however, endorsed and actively promoted by the National Empowerment Centre, where Ed has developed a platform from which to speak on the place of supported education, supported work and supported housing in psychiatric rehabilitation. The place of people with experience both as professionals and consumers within mental health care systems, argues Ed, is vital if new life is to be born from the ashes of psychiatric experience.

We return in our fifth narrative, *Avalon*, to the UK, where Liz Davies is shocked to discover that a misdiagnosis of schizophrenia remains on her medical record 30 years on from the episode of social invalidation which led to her false imprisonment in a mental hospital. Liz roots this political encounter firmly in the context of her family dynamics and the cultural milieu of the 1960s. Her account is a testimony to the long-term devastating effect of psychiatric labelling, but is also an indictment of the medical approach's inadequacy in discriminating between madness and mystical experience or in distinguishing between the two as separate components of an experience. Liz describes, in contrast with the psychiatric oppression she encountered, a truly spiritual sanctuary for those experiencing emotional turmoil, psychiatric emergency or spiritual emergence, on an island off the West Coast of Scotland owned by Tibetan Buddhists. In a long-established meditation cave on the island, used as a spiritual retreat for centuries, Liz recovers, writes out and to some extent resolves her experience.

We visit Australia a second and final time for our sixth piece, *A Most Precious Thread*, in which Simon Champ describes how he has managed, through decades of psychiatric care, obstinately to maintain communication with himself as to the meaning of his changing experience of psychosis and its treatment. A paradox is evident between reason and unreason here. Simon teases out methodically the personal meaning for him of gender and vocation, even recasting his sense of being in a psychiatric concentration camp, during an early admission, as no more than paranoia. Yet he is in no doubt as to the healing power of having such perceptions taken seriously and validated. If, in pathologizing his own experience thus, he is simply identifying with the oppressor, as he suspects, he nevertheless acknowledges that in the most important sense there is no ultimate reality beyond that which we construct for ourselves. The importance in this context of holding on to a thread of meaning and of establishing community is clear.

In the seventh narrative, *Hope, Humanity and Voice in Recovery from Mental Illness*, Dan Fisher, our final male contributor, does not explicitly deal with gender. Nevertheless, the poetry and inspirational quality of his writing, as well as the wonderful metaphors in his psychotic experience, certainly challenge any stereotypical notion of what might be expected from a man in a position of seniority and power. As a psychiatrist and Director of the National Empowerment Centre in the USA, Dan's assertion that a neurobiological theory of mental illness is disempowering, dehumanizing and ultimately unhelpful appears to carry some weight. But the strength of this piece probably derives mostly from the succinctness and poetry of Dan's writing and the call, once again, for greater humanity before any other considerations in improving mental health care. As a crucial facet in such re-humanized systems of care, instilling in people hope at least that they might find a voice – and therefore some meaning for their experience – is again prioritized.

We re-cross the Atlantic again to London in our eighth piece, *My Three Psychiatric Careers*, where Rachel Perkins contrasts the earlier overviews of what place spirituality might take in an ideal mental health system with a grounded account of her own encounter with bipolar affective disorder – manic depression. As much as any of our contributors, Rachel accepts the place of psychiatric medication to stabilize her mood swings, and more than any of them she extols the virtues of the medical model to help understand what is happening to her. Perhaps most importantly, Rachel distinguishes between the *perspective* and the *power* of psychiatry, returning ever to themes of interpersonal power, choice and the politics of diagnosis. Perhaps without meaning to, she embraces the spiritual themes more explicit elsewhere in the text when she asserts her right to pursue the life path and work ethic that has *meaning* for her, even if it ever were to prove a significant factor in her cycles of mental ill-health. In the meantime, Rachel's account of her synthesis of three careers in the mental health system – senior clinician, writer/campaigner and patient – complements not only Jan Holloway's parallel struggle but the themes running throughout the text of the symmetry and shared ground between the roles of professional and consumer in the mental health system.

We stay in the UK for our next piece, *Que Serà Serà*. Rose Snow's view could not be more different. Whatever her condition was, she echoes Liz Davies's insistence that a diagnosis of mental illness was worse than mistaken, it was anathema to her spirit. She did not need psychotropic poisoning, but help in integrating an experience of spiritual emergence following traumatic loss of her spiritual guide. Rose's description of the parallel journeys she has made – contending with both psychiatry and a psychic awakening – offers a stark account of the exhausting nature of the struggles probably all of our contributors have encountered. The resolution of Rose's anger at the psychiatrist cast as villain of her piece, and the strength of her personal resurrection – both in terms of her new careers and in terms of her growth through the experiences described – are testimony to the evolutionary potential inherent in what is called mental illness, however much scepticism one retains regarding the notion of spiritual reality.

In the tenth and final narrative, *The Medical Model and Harm*, Judi Chamberlin, our last contributor from the USA, reminds us of the way ordinary human experience, for example the natural distress occasioned by traumatic circumstances, can be pathologized and controlled, with the person experiencing it left, as a result of their treatment at the hands of psychiatry, feeling as though there is something *wrong with them*. In a series of logical steps Judi walks the reader through a brief but harrowing account of the way her grief became illness, her illness in turn a chronic psychiatric problem. Judi's anger at this process, always somewhere near the surface, was of course then further pathologized. We think this is a fitting finale to the accounts preceding it, a reminder of the central complaint of many of the contributors to this text about psychiatry, about which Judi does not mince her words: helping 'people to experience ... their pain, to grow and to heal is a far different enterprise, one that is about freedom, not control. And mental hospitals were not built to set people free.'

The concluding chapter is written by the editors and offers a review of the narratives and a summary of their implications for psychiatric and psychological theory-building in general, and the education of the major professional disciplines in mental health: medicine, nursing, psychotherapy, psychology, social work.

For generations it has been assumed that the stories told by people in mental distress are somehow inaccurate, flawed or downright invalid. The role of psychiatry has been to judge the validity of patients' accounts and to correct them, via therapy. A prevailing problem even of 'modern' psychiatry has been its reluctance to accept stories such as those we have collected for this text as valuable in their own right. Traditionally, the patient's story only becomes meaningful once it has been interpreted, or otherwise explicated, through the psychiatric process. In contrast, here we are pleased to offer stories that are both complete and unfinished at one and the same time. As MacQuarrie (1973, p. 78) noted:

> The fact that man [sic] is unfinished and on his way does not mean that a description is impossible, but that such a description should be directed to possibilities rather than properties.

In that sense the reader may be interested in what the stories tell us of the *becoming* of the people involved. We recognize that the storytellers are the story. Their uniqueness and unfinished status is their strength.

The forms of language in our contributors' various stories manifest a powerful force. Through language we construct our world. The stories told by our authors and the language they employ serve as a means by which they have been able to construct and describe their own world-as-they-conceive-it, and tell their own, not psychiatry's or anyone else's story. They have all long since abandoned the notion that what they experience is an affliction. We hope that the reader may, through reading these accounts, share a more sensitive appreciation of the total reality of the 'madness experience', its politics and its potential for growth.

Phil Barker, Peter Campbell and Ben Davidson, June 1999

Reference

MacQuarrie J (1973) 20th Century Religious Thought: The Frontiers of Philosophy and Theology. London: SCM Press.

Acknowledgements

We would like to express our gratitude to Dr Irene Whitehill for her many helpful comments on the early drafts of the book, and to Dr Liz Davies for allowing us to use her illustration of the Phoenix taken from *The Firebird* published by Firebird Press.

Chapter 1
Introduction

PHIL BARKER, PETER CAMPBELL AND BEN
DAVIDSON

The Swampy Lowlands of Human Experience

At some point in our history, in the moment when we moved, according to
Western Buddhist thought, from our biological evolution into an early
stage of the *Higher Evolution,* people became aware that they were aware.
In that moment of illumination, as a prehistoric prelude to what Jaspers
(1953) has called *the Axial Age,* a person's experience of something
unusual or mundane was held for the first time in reflexive consciousness.

In the time it took to register one person's appreciation of an unusual
experience, whether it was an experience of a novel idea about the world
around her or simply the experience of herself *as an experiencing being,* an
awareness of discomfiting individuality and difference, the concept of
madness too, were probably born. In that moment lay the origins of the
dis-ease with which we continue to struggle millions of years later. It is a
dis-ease that remains bound up in the personal histories of people struggling with their 'experience of experience'.

If alien anthropologists police our skies they may wonder what all the
fuss is about. For a long, long time, *Homo Sapiens* has appreciated that just
about everything obeys a certain law of averages: the science of statistics
has enshrined this effect in the 'Gaussian curve', a graphic representation
of the way that, with most phenomena, a main cluster of data will emerge
around a mean point, with some results falling evenly either side of the
mean, and a still smaller number of extreme outliers distributed either side
of the vast majority. This curve is the shape of a rounded, steeply sloping
hill, or a bell jar; hence the pop-scientific term for this phenomenon: *'the
bell-jar effect'.* For example, at the extremes of such a curve, if it were to
represent the intelligence of a large group of people, would lie the highly
intelligent and those of limited intelligence. At the wider extremes still

would be geniuses and those with severe learning difficulties. Most people would lie under the main, bulging section of the curve, in the middle. At any point in history and in relation to almost any phenomenon, nearly all people will have been found under the bell jar curve, with only small minorities occupying its outlying reaches – those who deviate furthest from the norm. In most such cases their deviance from the norm is regarded as of largely statistical significance. But madness, we are encouraged to believe, is unlike any other human experience or characteristic. The mad are an alien people, beyond the pale, people who have crossed some invisible boundary, and now we gaze at them as if they were literally from another world. It is as though the bell jar was taken from the realm of science and statistics, the glass melted down, and a normative lens constructed from it, through which we look in judgement on those veering too far from the statistical norm. The construction of those experiencing mental illness in the Nazi realm as 'Lebensunwerten Lebens' ('lives not worthy of living') and 'Ballastexistenzen' ('human ballast') (Binding and Hocke, 1920) represents a difference in degree, not in kind, from Western society's ordinary construction of such people.

All those years ago, when our ancestor became aware of some new experience – of the world in contrast with that which might be outside it; of 'self' in contrast with 'other'; of circularity as an abstract ideal; or of combustion as a process which might be harnessed – the simple act of communicating something of that experience to the rest of the group must have been threatening. Perhaps those others had not yet appreciated the exquisite freedom and terrifying isolation of individual selfhood, or the unique qualities of a round stone rolling down a hill; they had perhaps not yet come to appreciate the special taste of boar, left toasting in the heat of the fire. Perhaps they had not yet visualized their world in two-dimensional form, in the eye of the mind, as an image that could be projected to the walls of the cave with a burnt twig, or with a dry stick and some wet earth. And our evolving ancestor might herself not easily have found the words or the confidence to communicate any of these things. Although these discoveries have to be recapitulated again and again as each child struggles to evolve its consciousness, all those years ago minds were just beginning to be acquired and self-awareness was even more primitive than now. When a member of the group had a sudden and unexpected experience of mind stretching, the message must have sounded strange and exciting, but mostly strange and daunting. Down the millennia little has changed. Whenever a member of today's pack experiences a bit of mind stretching beyond the strictly limited type expected in normal development, a common response is often one of fascination and excitement, certainly, but more often one of apprehension and threat – 'what is going on (in their head) and where might it lead to?'

The alien anthropologist is dumbfounded. *Homo Sapiens* manages to journey to the stars, walking with his own feet on the face of the moon and plumbing the depths of the ocean. *Homo Sapiens* unravels the mysteries of the structure of physical life, even developing a telescope to look backwards through the universe to the possible dawn of time itself. However, *Homo Sapiens* remains afraid of experiences that lie just at the edge of the bell jar curve. We have travelled far in our journey from our primal roots to near-bionic status. But Eliot (1959) may have known *Homo Sapiens* better than most when he observed that:

> We shall not cease from exploration
> And the end of our exploring
> Will be to arrive where we started
> And know the place again for the first time.

(p. 148)

Perhaps we have spent all this time journeying, first from the swamp to the solid ground, and then out into space, so that we might return to the swamp of our primitive fears and know the place again for the first time.

Tour Guides and Black Holes

This book is an addition to a huge literature that describes our repeated visits to that primitive place where first our ancestors glimpsed, felt, sensed or otherwise experienced something 'different'.

Much of that literature can be seen as one or another form of tour guide, some highly articulate, methodical, respectful and well researched, others of small literary value, blinkered, unashamedly xenophobic and ill-informed. In either case though, they appear to be tour guides designed not so much for those who might themselves visit such places as for those who have an interest in understanding, in the absence of any such journey, how to deal with, treat or otherwise manage someone from that place. They describe from the outside the prominent features of the landscape. They classify the commonly occurring patterns of behaviour, thought, emotion and relationship, and advance interesting – but often prepos-terous – interpretations as to the cause, role, function and meaning of such phenomena. They conjure up fascinating titles, labels and synonyms for grouping some of them together.

It is obvious that the existence, for some travellers, of such psychiatric manuals, textbooks and other such tour guides is useful. If nothing leads you to value the journey, if you have run out of resources and simply want the embassy to return you safely home so you can forget as quickly as possible that you ever entertained such a hare-brained scheme as to travel (if indeed it was ever planned), such guides may be more than sufficient. You would not want to read them yourself but, if they are well prepared, they do occasionally (although perhaps less often than professionals like to think) offer the outsider a useful way of getting to know something of the road system of that foreign terrain from which they will help you, their unhappy compatriot, return. The tour guide does help attach names to phenomena in the landscape and gain some appreciation of the overall scene. And depending on your proclivity for experiencing the world via reason, emotion, ethics or corporeality, one or another of these tour guides might even encourage you to develop some understanding and familiarity with the route home.

Throughout the short history of the creation of these tour guides, the industry has been unsettled by fierce and proprietorial polemic focused on the extent to which one or another form of tour guide can tell us, or other outsiders, how to manage the unfortunate traveller's absence and return. Although travel by sea, air and land may all be appropriate at some point of the journey, the proponents of each are often blinkered as to the merits of the others.

These arguments seem set to proliferate as the neuroscientists, their eye ever and only on the material realm, sharpen their saw. *Homo Sapiens* is not wise in the human terms we once understood in our romantic past. *Homo Sapiens* is only a clever machine, genetically determined and, in sapiential terms, ultimately meaningless. Indeed, mental illness, long considered to be a gross affliction of the mind, may soon be dismissed from our history by erasing the original concept of mind. Francis Crick who, along with James Watson, described the structure of DNA, has pontificated on the essential structure of human experience, arguing that all human joys, sorrows, memories and ambitions, sense of personal identity and free will, 'the you that is you ... is in fact no more than the behaviour of a vast assembly of nerve cells and their associated molecules' (Crick, 1994, p. 3).

Doctors of the soul, the shamans and priests of old, once attributed the complexities of human experience to the influence of abstract, invisible forces. Their most powerful counterparts today, neuroscientists, are on the brink of reversing that age-old rule about babies and bath water. They want to keep the bath water, for they can, metaphorically, test its proper-ties. The baby is, however, quite different, and clearly has to go – all that meaningless crying strains the scientific ear.

But let us return to our various visitors and their quests to foreign soil. It is obvious that an English Egyptologist has a quite different experience of that country from even the poorest, least travelled Egyptian. The native senses in his very body are in connection with forces the outsider can only imagine. The Egyptian feels a connection either with the Pharaohs, or with the slaves who built their pyramids, quite beyond the experience of the Egyptologist, let alone a foreign office official dispatched to bring his countryman home.

This book is not a tour guide in any of the distant and distancing styles described; rather it is a collection of stories of people who have found their journeyings in foreign territory valuable and want to share the experiences they have encountered, particularly experiences of rediscovering their own map, finding their own way to a destination of their own choosing, knowing again for the first time and knowing well that place where they started, and wanting to help others who feel lost.

The Wisdom of Uncertainty and the Refuge of Insecurity

An appreciation of what it is like authentically to be-in-the-world – especially an appreciation of impermanence or that death is inevitable, that life might be meaningless, that we have no ultimate essence and are ultimately free to do as we wish, or that we die, just as we live, ultimately alone – frequently sends us scurrying in search of a model, or a theory, which will lend security and stability to our shaken selves. The empty certainties of neuroscience, or the playful structures of 101 forms of cogni-tive, behavioural and psychodynamic therapy, are like a salve for our anxious souls. Indeed, our theorizing, especially when it takes some of the more concrete cause and effect forms, does away with the soul, and with it any need for human anxiety.

In this respect, the psychiatric knowledge we have developed, especially within this century, is little different from an ideological security blanket. Instead of representing an advance for the human race, our blind faith in science diminishes us:

> We say we are reasonable men, but we accept the pronouncement of our
> scientists with a faith quite as grovelling as the faith of peasants who

believe unquestioningly those who say they have seen gods or demons.
How many people could prove such common beliefs as that the earth
revolves around the sun or that atoms are composed of electrons and
protons. (Watts, 1978, p. 76)

We might well ask, in the same vein, to what extent any of us, patient or
professional, really know what we are talking about when we repeat
mindlessly the medical mantras which pass for an explanation of the
experience labelled manic depression or schizophrenia.

It used to be a commonplace to observe that psychiatrists were as mad
as their patients. Regrettably, perhaps, that old music hall routine no
longer rings true. Psychiatrists and all their mental health fellow travellers
tend, nowadays, to be all too normal. They grip their weighty tour guides
to their chests and feel the security of their classificatory systems, their
clinical protocols and their evidence-based quality standards. It may well
be true that they have no real lived experience of madness, but, after all,
you do not need to have had pneumonia to be able to treat it. In possession
of this corporate intelligence, the mental health worker might sit back and
enjoy the trip, alongside her patient, to that place which they might know
again together for the first time; or, then again, she might not.

In an interview with the actor Mark Rylance, who was one of the
Royal Shakespeare Company which brought Shakespeare, under the
auspices of the late Murray Cox, to Broadmoor,[3] Rob Ferris the psychiatrist commented:

> There is a workaday sense in which we look at people's experiences and try
> to categorise them fairly crudely and bluntly as normal or abnormal, as part
> of the process of diagnosing mental illness and deciding about treatment.
> Perhaps it might be said that this process actively avoids the spiritual aspects
> or dimension which something like the play taps. (Ferris, 1992, p. 33)

This touched a nerve in Rylance, prompting him to consider the process of
coming to understand the irrational in some of Shakespeare's characters:

> Perhaps that's why there are so many books written about Hamlet; yet
> none of them could explain what some of the lines meant. It took me 80 or
> 90 performances before I learned what some of them meant. There is no

---

[3] Broadmoor is one of three Special Hospitals in the UK for the care and control of the
criminally insane. The consultant psychotherapist Murray Cox invited the RSC to put
on Shakespeare's work there in the late 1980s, with patients participating in the
productions.

way you can do it with a dictionary or rational thought. It is only through play that you get there. (Ferris, 1992, p. 33)

This conversation, between a professional actor and a psychiatrist, revealed two extraordinary truths: the psychiatric process appears to be predicated on shying away from the human condition; and the only way to appreciate the real meaning of human distress is to imagine oneself into the experience, even enacting it, somehow playing it out to appreciate its significance.

To court such familiarity with madness as their conversation seems to prescribe may be to disarm oneself of the protective cover of our imagined knowledge, but it might also lead us to a more authentic appreciation of the human experience behind the 'illness' and a more genuine claim to occupy the Shaman role, walking alongside the 'ill' person in their euphoria, turmoil, hatred or despair.

The Politics of Madness

The question then arises as to why we find it so hard as individuals, professions, groups, to acknowledge and validate the experience of those who find their way into the psychiatric system. But perhaps the question should be reversed:

> Given the ascendancy of a scientific, empirical view of reality wherein subjective experience is generally either devalued or invalidated completely, both [the 'mentally ill'] and those treating them find it hard not to succumb to pressures to accept the conventional wisdom. In these circumstances, it is much easier to call experiential suffering and its results 'illness' and treat them as such. (Davidson, 1998, p. 59)

People's experience and subjective world seem often, by the time they reach the realm of mental health professionals, to have been so devastated that one:

> ...often find[s] it too awful and dismaying to want to explore it. The *act of faith* [required] seems at such times to be more a plunge into the abyss. (Davidson, 1998, p. 62)

It is virtually impossible to consider the *meaning* of madness without considering the deployment by society of a psychiatric gaze and the complex politics of labelling (Foucault, 1971). Who the mentally ill *are* cannot be separated from the interests of the community legitimizing and justifying a social relationship of control and exclusion (Jodelet, 1991, p. 298). One of the arch-critics of anti-psychiatry, Peter Sedgwick, attempted to dismiss mental illness as no more than another form of *deviancy* and, in that sense, no different from physical illness, which also represents a deviation from the norm. However, Sedgwick's (1982) critique failed to acknowledge the key feature of madness: it is a whole human experience. Whereas a person *has* pneumonia or cancer, he *is* mentally distressed or mad – the person and the madness appear to be one and the same. The central importance of the *experience* may well be the feature of madness which so terrifies those who view themselves as normal. Becker drew a similar conclusion 25 years ago, suggesting that psychotic people expose the fragile self-esteem of others:

> The manic seems to make a frantic bid for ... power and succeeds ... in creating massive discomfort; the depressed person actually shows up our whole social ceremonial by choosing to opt out of it. Probably the most troublesome illness of all, from a ceremonial point of view, is the person who renounces all zest for life in the game we are so dedicatedly playing; it unnerves us that someone can be so indifferent to everything we cherish. (Becker, 1972, pp. 139–140)

Much of our contemporary fascination with what is happening in the deeper structures of the brain and its biochemistry can be read as an elaborate defence against recognizing that the most disturbing feature of madness is not biological, but ceremonial. Goffman (1956) noted how the gradations of 'mental illness', at least in hospital, reflected the degree to which patients violated ceremonial rules of social intercourse (p. 497). In Becker's view, people 'who are the least ready to project a sustainable self' unnerve and disorientate so-called 'normals':

> The mentally ill – indeed everyone we care to call abnormal, has in some way touched us at times, and in places where we do not feel it proper to be touched. (p. 140)

It seems that in this book we have taken such political considerations as our starting and end-point. We should never forget how the bestowal of a psychiatric label can so usurp the person's sense of identity that all subsequent distress (relapse) is reconstructed as a function of that diagnosis (Szasz, 1974). We are obstinate in recalling how the scientific pretensions and rhetoric of psychiatry belie its ceremonial role in the politics of interpersonal experience:

My first crisis admission was not a medical event. For me, it was a moral
event, a moral failure. All my subsequent admissions have contained
shadows of that first failure. None of the important implications have been
medical ones. (Campbell, 1996, p. 57)

The way psychiatry succeeds, nevertheless, in informing and influencing
our view of madness is central to this text.

In contrast, and in our efforts to develop a truly *human* craft of psychiatry, we begin with the stories of people in various forms of mental
distress, and we end up perhaps by finding some of ourselves *in* those
stories; and some of that distress *in* ourselves. These may be dismissed as
no more than echoes, or even heightened empathy, but for many of us
those echoes of our own tiny voice can still be too much to bear, prompting
us to turn away, or develop another way of responding 'therapeutically'.

Although we three share some kind of consensus as to the human
context of madness and mental distress, we shrink from the suggestion that
we speak with one voice. We are still too much involved in discovering one
another, and ourselves, to have reached that degree of certainty. Although
we may be more alike than different, how far this is true of the other
contributors is less clear. Given that they come from differing cultures,
backgrounds and ends of the earth, this is unremarkable. By the end of this
book the reader will, hopefully, be fascinated by that place which has been
revisited, albeit perhaps vicariously, and may have come to appreciate a
very personal, and hopefully more democratic kind of knowledge of
mental illness as a result.

The March of Ignorance

It is tempting to assume that humankind has been making sustained
progress down the ages. Technology advances certainly, but what of our
understanding of ourselves, of our experiences, of one another? Although
there are now, literally, hundreds of names for mental distress (or illness)
the knowledge of lay people remains primitive. Perhaps they have an in-
built resistance to understanding madness, or perhaps there is a more
sinister agenda, encouraging a culture of misinformation, and the creation
of 'moral panics' involving the mentally ill (Barker et al., 1998a).

As we wrote this introduction, two British newspapers carried reports
about people with mental illness. Both newspapers are commonly
regarded as liberal organs, with a liberal-minded and educated readership.

One might assume that these newspapers would inform further the informed minority. The 'Tuesday Review' in *The Independent* carried a lengthy feature about Michael Laudor:

> ...a schizophrenic who battled with his demons and won. Hollywood paid
> $1.5m for his story; Brad Pitt was going to play him. But a tale of triumph
> over adversity has become a horror story. Michael Laudor cracked, and
> stabbed his pregnant girlfriend to death. (Usborne, 1998)

Two days later the same newspaper carried a headline detailing the abuse of 'mentally ill' people in a residential home. The story revealed that the people were in fact suffering from a learning disability, with the 'mental ages of young children'. *The Independent*'s editor added insult to injury by writing an editorial bemoaning the woeful standard of care offered to 'vulnerable' 'mentally ill' people. Some days later, a representative of a national learning disability charity pointed out in the letters column the difference between mental illness and mental handicap. After all the public information campaigns, the explosion of books, films and plays featuring people with various forms of mental illness and handicap, the (educated) journalists and editor of a broadsheet remain trapped by their ignorance.

A few weeks later, *The Guardian* – another liberal broadsheet with a reputation for quality journalism – carried a feature on the killing of a woman by a young man who had been described as 'psychotic', but who also had a history of communication difficulties, deafness and, by implication, learning difficulties. The actual events seemed in themselves to have been sufficiently melodramatic. This did not deter the author from adding his own piece of journalistic spice to the story, suggesting that the killing could be explained by the young man having stopped taking his medication:

> Daniel ... turned to the Lord and stopped taking his Risperidone. Disaster
> was only two months away. The pharmaceutical plug which had held back
> his illness started to dissolve, and the psychosis leaked back into his
> system. (Davies, 1998, p. 3)

Later in the feature the author reports, with a complete absence of irony, that a National Confidential Inquiry into Suicide and Homicide by People with Mental Illness revealed that '12 per cent of homicides and 26 per cent of suicides are committed by people who are mentally ill'. Although these deaths may have been preventable, given alternative care and treatment provisions, an informed society needs to keep such statistics in perspective. The figures betray the more frightening statistic that people are at greater risk from (so-called) 'normal' people, than from the 'mentally ill'. Since most mentally ill (even psychotic) people are patently more vulnerable than dangerous, why do public information organs continue to promote the traditional myth that the 'psychotic' is dangerous or that horrendous killings can be explained simply by 'psychosis leaking back into [someone's] system.'

We appear to comfort ourselves with two facts: the mentally ill are an alien species but a simple remedy is available to transform them into close approximations of normal humans. The alien anthropologist may be bewildered at this point, having realized that, as Western civilization reaches its zenith, the faith system which underpins psychiatry remains crude, if not obviously fallacious.

No less an authority than Einstein recognized the witlessness of blind faith in science, especially when applied beyond its limits. When he was asked: 'Do you believe that absolutely everything can be expressed scientifically?' he replied:

> Yes, it would be possible, but it would make no sense. It would be a description without meaning as if you described a Beethoven symphony as a variation of wave pressure. (Knudtson and Suzuki, 1997, p. 65)

In one important sense, Einstein affirms the importance of *awe*. Some things are simply beyond explanation – or at least *meaningful* explanation. However, we may have long since passed the point in our human development where we can still feel comfortable with uncertainty; can still marvel and wonder, especially about aspects of the human condition.

The Ordinariness of Mad Experience

Despite their efforts, we suspect that today's armies of mental health workers – psychiatrists, psychiatric nurses, psychologists, psychotherapists, occupational therapists and social workers – are not as ordinary and functional as they paint themselves. We suspect that they have merely acquired great competence in representing themselves in this way. If we did not wish to avoid giving ourselves away too much, we might even say that such calmness in the face of manifest human distress is a *defence*: a basic mechanism to avoid recognizing something which cries out for recognition.

Freud's work has been largely dismissed as hocus-pocus, mumbo-jumbo, or (worst of all) unverifiable – and therefore bad science. Yet the enigmatic object of his attention – how madness is woven, invisibly, into the warp and woof of our lives – remains. It has become unfashionable to suggest that we might *all* be in some sense possessed of madness; or somehow be holding it, like a sleeping giant, in check, deep within us. Instead, we have returned to the age-old 'us-and-them' mentality and morality, which Freud began to dislodge a century ago. Perhaps that simple gesture – the recognition of his own human failing – was the greatest contribution that he made.

Fifty years ago, Harry Stack Sullivan, like Jung before him, threw away Freud's original rule book, and immersed himself in intense relationships with people in psychosis: those whom Freud had allowed to remain beyond the human pale. In those relationships Sullivan was also to confront *himself*, as Freud had done with his neurotic patients. In the company of people in the severest forms of psychosis Sullivan discovered for himself that we are all much more simply human than otherwise. People who are patients and people who intend to become their therapeutic guides have much more in common than many would care to admit. In the words of the old Scottish adage, we are all Jock Tamson's bairns – we all belong to the family of (wo)man; we are all more alike than different.

Sullivan appeared to be one of the first psychiatrists, at least in modern times, to challenge the orthodoxy of defining and developing *psychiatric diagnoses*, preferring instead to talk of people's *'difficulties in living'*. More importantly, he was one of the first psychiatrists to acknowledge publicly (to his biographer and colleagues) that he had experienced a schizophrenic state, and been hospitalized in Bellevue Hospital (Evans, 1996). Ironically, the courage of those particular convictions appears to have played a significant part in the widespread dismissal of Sullivan's work, following his early death in 1949.

Sullivan's influence reappeared in the early 1960s in the work of R. D. Laing, who pursued a similar interest in the experience of psychosis from a devout existential perspective and who was more concerned with the interpersonal space and the *politics* of experience therein, than any 'inner reality' (Kotowicz, 1997). Laing's early fame and his descent into infamy have been all too widely reported. His downfall, like Sullivan's, appeared to pivot around his personal proximity to psychosis and distress. Although his legacy is tarnished, the rise of the self-help movement in Britain (in particular) bears a direct imprint of his work. The Mental Patients Union (MPU) established in 1973, and later Survivors Speak Out, reflected the need for, and value of, organized forms of *ownership* of the psychiatric experience. Although these two groups (and the journal *Asylum*) have often taken an unashamed anti-psychiatric line, not all the authors in this text would necessarily share this position. Indeed, Alex Jenner, the editor of *Asylum* and Emeritus Professor of Psychiatry at Sheffield (arguably also the only senior British psychiatrist to take seriously the question of patients' rights), could never be called an anti-psychiatrist. He is, nevertheless, a humanitarian. This text is focused on the humanitarian response to madness, and the human experience that lies at its heart.

Through a Glass Darkly

It is hoped that this book will serve as a mirror for the readership, which risks finding something of itself in the act of reading the authors' reflections on themselves. It may bring out something of the similarity between the reader and the author. The act of reading may promote understanding, but perhaps it may also sensitize readers to their ignorance, uncertainty and fear. It may allow some of us not to feel so alone with our own fear, and others of us not to feel so distant from the experiences described that we sit in judgement of our patients. Whatever the reaction, the act of *engaging* with these stories should be meaningful.

In this sense the text – the collection of narratives and reflections – becomes like a work of fiction. We may learn a great deal about ourselves by reading the life stories of others, which blend the authors' personal truths with concurrent reflection in the manner of many a great novel. The authors did not set out to help individual readers approach and clarify their own demons. That ambitious aim was, however, part of our (at least covert) agenda. One key to unlocking a more compassionate and caring mental health care system might be the development of some awareness of the potential wounded healer status of all mental health workers (Barker et al., 1998b).

Our aim is thus educational in origin: we hope that the experience of reading will draw out (educe) something of the reader's own experience. In that kind of educational context Joyce suggested that his intention in writing *Dubliners* was 'to advance civilisation in Ireland' by giving the Irish people 'one good look at themselves in [his] nicely-polished looking glass' (McCarthy, 1990). The *Dubliners* of the title were both the characters and those who were reading about the characters.

Given a similarly reciprocal nature to the relationships determining our readers' experience of our authors' experience, we hope the text may rekindle interest in what it means to *be* mentally ill (or mad, or distressed) as distinct from the experience of *having* such a phenomenon. In Fromm's (1993) view we have taken too long a walk down the *having* route. Although we cannot exist without *having*, much of what we *have* is useless, or makes life difficult.

Perhaps the idea that people might 'have' mental illness, rather than 'be' mad, might have contributed to the denial of that curious form of journeying and growing through life that madness can represent.

And, in the final analysis, for some of the authors at least, the understanding reached so far has a spiritual quality. The stories are of journeys, and the roads taken have often been test beds for the mettle of the individual. The stories may even be a kind of prayer, or at least a genuflection before that which shapes our human destinies: experience.

William Johnston, the Irish Jesuit, recognized that the core of existential prayer is analogous to journey:

> At first your journey may go smoothly ... but sooner or later you will run into turbulence. But the time must come when you hit a major crisis, which is like an earthquake shaking you to the roots of your being. Such an upheaval may occur two or three times in a lifetime. It is a turning point, a time of growth, and it is important that you recognise it as such. (Johnston, 1989, p. 83)

If these stories are not all forms of prayer then, at least, all of them must be seen as closely connected to the conscience of the author. We hope they will connect with the conscience of the reader, for, as Marcuse believed:

> A radical change in consciousness is the necessary first step towards radical social change. (1974, p. 121)

References

Barker P, Croom S, Stevenson C, Adam T, Reynolds B (1998a) Serious mental illness: modern myths and grim realities. Journal of Psychiatric and Mental Health Nursing 5(4): 247–254.

Barker P, Manos E, Novak V, Reynolds B (1998b) The wounded healer and the myth of mental well-being: ethical issues concerning the mental health status of psychiatric nurses. In Barker P, Davidson B (Eds) Psychiatric Nursing: Ethical Strife. London: Arnold, pp 334–348.

Becker E (1972) The Birth and Death of Meaning. Harmondsworth: Penguin.

Binding K, Hoche S (1920) Die Freigabe der Vernichtung Lebensunwerten Lebens (The granting of permission for the destruction of worthless life. Its extent and form). Leipzig.

Campbell P (1996) Challenging loss of power. In Read J, Reynolds J (Eds) Speaking Our Minds: An Anthology. London: Macmillan/Open University Press.

Crick F (1994) The Astonishing Hypothesis. New York: Simon & Schuster.

Davidson B (1998) The role of the psychiatric nurse. In Barker P, Davidson B, Psychiatric Nursing: Ethical Strife. London: Arnold, pp 57–65.

Davies N (1998) System failure. The Guardian (G2), 14 July.

Eliot TS (1959) 'Little Gidding' in Four Quartets, Faber and Faber.

Evans FB (1996) Harry Stack Sullivan: Interpersonal Theory and Psychotherapy. London: Routledge.

Ferris R (1992) Hamlet and Romeo: Mark Rylance. In Cox M (Ed) Shakespeare Comes to Broadmoor. London: Jessica Kingsley.

Foucault M (1971) Madness and Civilisation. London: Tavistock.

Fromm E (1993) The Art of Being. London: Constable.

Goffman E (1956) The nature of difference and demeanor. American Anthropologist 58: 495–498.

Jaspers K (1953) The origin and goal of history. New Haven, CT: Yale University Press.

Jodelet D (1991) Madness and Social Representation: Living with the Mad in a French Community. Berkeley: University of California Press.

Johnston W (1989) Being in Love: The Practice of Christian Prayer. London: Fount Paperbacks.

Knudtson P, Suzuki D (1997) Wisdom of the Elders. St Leonards, NSW: Allen & Unwin.

Kotowicz Z (1997) RD Laing and the Paths of Anti-Psychiatry. London: Routledge.

Marcuse H (1974) Eros and Civilisation: A Philosophical Inquiry into Freud. Boston: Beaumont.

McCarthy J (1990) Ulysses – Portals of Discovery. Boston: Twayne Publishers.

Sedgwick P (1982) Psycho-Politics. London: Pluto Press.

Szasz TS (1974) Ideology and Insanity. Harmondsworth: Penguin.

Usborne D (1998) The two faces of Michael. The Independent 23 June.

Watts A (1978) The Meaning of Happiness. London: Rider (original edition 1940).

Chapter 2
Madness and Reality

Sally Clay

Editorial

Sally's is a house of many mansions. She encourages the reader to see beyond the simple notion of a healthy person who falls ill, in favour of asking what is the true nature and function of the experience of 'falling' out of the consensual reality. Sally pursues that question in several ways: What is the nature of madness? Why does it appear to hold, for some, the secrets of consciousness, of healing and of spiritual power? What is its link to the visions and prophetic experiences described in the Old Testament? How do people recover wellness as opposed to merely coping? And what, indeed, is wellness, or recovery? All these questions are stimulated by a profound experience, which begins with enlighten-ment and turns to despair. Sally Clay takes the reader along some of the pathways she needed to take to recover sight of that enlightenment. Her story is a fine example of the road less travelled.

Sally Clay's journey in and out of the various altered states commonly called madness brought her into contact with an archaic psychiatric system in the 1950s, and into contact with many others who fared less well with such experiences. Those people reflected the harsh wisdom of the saying that 'the illness was successfully treated, but the patient died in the process'. What Sally saw repeatedly was a death of the spirit, something that she strove to avoid.

Sally Clay's journey ended, at least temporarily, in a community where the workers, led by an enlightened psychiatrist, aimed for understanding of madness, whilst appreciating that the promise of revelation is an experience that can seduce the person. Like all seductions, this can be attractive, but might ultimately involve loss, if only a loss of a place in the ordinary world. Here lies the great challenge for mental health workers, who believe that, after years of devoted study, they have emerged with some knowledge that might be used to 'help' their clientele. Sally Clay's story reminds us of the unfocused, if not completely off-beam, nature of much psychiatric knowledge. Knowledge of the meaning of pilgrimage through dimensions of consciousness and practice of spiritual disciplines to enhance wisdom and compassion may be more important tools for psychiatry to help its clientele to transact the recovery process. Or, as Sally points out, perhaps recovery is the wrong way of looking at what happens when people emerge from the transformation of madness.

$\star \quad \star \quad \star \quad \star \quad \star$

First Institution

When I came to, I was sitting at the corner of a grimy wooden table. At the other end two dishevelled women slumped over the table staring at their hands and feet, shaking uncontrollably. Sitting in the shadows against the wall were eight or nine other women. One or two of them seemed young like me; the others were of an indeterminate age. None of them talked to each other; only a few attempted mumbling sounds. Several had slipped down in their chairs with legs spread, asleep.

The few windows near the ceiling had bars that blocked out most of the light. The only door was on the other side of the room, and it was locked. The door had a scratched plastic window about eight inches square. On a shelf hanging from the ceiling was an old TV set. It was not turned on, and it was placed so that none of the people in the room could reach it. Later I learned that it did not even work. There were no other furnishings in the room, and there was nothing to do there except to sit and soak up the gloom and the stench from old urine.

A feeling of cold horror grew inside me. I had awakened into a nightmare, deepened by a strange, soupy grogginess that made it difficult even to open my eyes or move my head. I felt an interior restlessness as if my internal organs were convulsing, although my external senses were paralysed. My mouth was dry and foul tasting, and I would have had a hard time speaking even if I had wanted to. I knew where I was. This was a mental hospital, the bottomless pit where society's refuse was thrown. As I examined this place I realized that for the first time in my life – perhaps now for all my life – I was identified with the lowest of the low. This was the hell that sophisticated people said did not exist. Was this really me sitting here?

As if in slow motion, and with great effort, I opened my hand close to my face to study the lines on my palm. I was relieved at least to recognize my own hand, my own blunt-tipped fingers and the familiar map of lines on my palm. My hand, too, was trembling like those of the other women – I pressed it down palm up on the table to ease the shaking, and tried to read my destiny there, to understand why I was in this place. Although my feelings, like my body, seemed cloaked in an enforced apathy, I tried to muster a protest. What was being done to me? What had happened to the astonishing brilliance and spiritual power that had been so real such a short time ago? Surely I should be receiving tender and respectful help rather than this degradation? I had seen a vision of the world transformed. How could something so precious be relegated to a place of the damned? Why? Why?

I do not know how long I sat staring at my hand, trying to reconcile the horror of this place with the fragile memories of my recent experience. At first I mourned the loss of my vision, that its truth had become ignominy, its hope shattered to misery. Had I made some terrible mistake that I was brought to this? Could it be that my encounter with spiritual energy meant nothing – or worse than nothing, that it was an empty and evil dream, and I was nothing but a fool? As my confidence in my spiritual experience faded, so did any belief in my own life and values. Unconsciously I began to believe that I was horribly wrong to find meaning in my experience, and that because of this, I could never again dare to dream, or even to hope for any good in my life. In one fell swoop, my mind grieved for and renounced my college studies, my career as a writer, my present and future worthiness, and my hope for any future happiness. It was all gone. In the space of a few minutes, I steeled myself to tolerate the requirements of living in this place. I had to learn to live in hell.

I sat in the same place for a long time, weeping numbly, for I could not make my mouth move and I could not produce tears. I could not see properly, for I had neither my contact lenses nor my glasses. The dryness of my mouth was almost palpable, like a stifled cry that cannot be swallowed. I found myself staring at the door until my eyes burned, waiting but hardly daring to hope that it would eventually be opened. Time passed and nothing happened. I had to go to the bathroom. Eventually I struggled to stand up – my legs and my arms hardly seemed to belong to me and responded faultily to my intents. I could not stand up straight and had to shuffle across the room grasping the edge of the table and the backs of chairs. Finally I reached the door and fumbled around its edge. There was no doorknob or handle of any kind. I ran my hand up and down the dark-green-painted wood; it was covered with random nicks and deliberate scratches around the edge where the doorknob should have been and around the cloudy window. I stood on tiptoe to look out of the window, and squinting at the featureless hall that was on the other side, took a deep breath. Oh God, please help me!

'Help!' I cried in a scratchy whisper. I tried again, 'Help!' but all that came out was a croak. I could not try any more, and sank exhausted into a chair by the door. There again I sat for a very long time. The room was getting darker and darker, so that I could not see much of anything, when at last a bare bulb in the centre of the ceiling flooded the room with harsh light, and I heard the sound of keys in the lock. The door burst open and three women in white stepped inside. 'Well, Sally,' said the first woman, surprised to see me in the chair, 'we've moved around today, haven't we?' I could only stare at her. I did not know who she was, and I had no way of knowing that I had already been in this place for some time and had spent many days immobile and unaware at the long table. I had been brought directly here after the medics brutally removed me from my room at Sarah Lawrence, and the shock of that experience literally paralysed me. Later the doctor would tell me that I had become totally catatonic and that he had feared that I would never come out of it.

But now I cowered before these three large women in white. The one who had spoken to me stood over me holding a tray full of miniature paper cups. Apparently unimpressed by my 'miraculous' improvement, she handed me one of these little cups and took a cup of water from one of the other women. 'Let's see if you can do this yourself today', she said briskly. In the cup was a pill that looked like an oversized brown M&M. 'What is this?' I tried to ask, but again all that came out of my lips was a bleat. I greedily drank the entire delicious cup of water, and tried again. 'What is this?'

'Take the pill, Sally', said the nurse impatiently. 'You can drink water with your dinner.' I did as I was told. The three women then moved around the room with no further comments. All of the other inmates received their pills, a few taking them with no assistance, others needing to be shaken awake, coaxed, or manually assisted. When they were finished the women left, locking the door behind them. I managed again to stand up to watch the retreating figures through the little window. I still had to go to the bathroom, but I now did not dare to call for help. I stood and waited. Inside the room the light bulb in the ceiling cast a dim but harsh light and equally harsh shadows, mercilessly laying bare the grey faces of the women there. They were, to me, the living dead, and although I knew that I was among them, I again protested. I did not belong here. This was wrong.

Not too much time passed before the nurses appeared again, and this time they opened the door wide. 'Dinner is ready!' one of them announced, and they began leading us out of our ill-lit cell and down the hallway, which was in comparison brightly bathed in yellow light. One of the nurses had gripped my arm and my side with steely fingers, and she was half-dragging, half-pushing me down the hall. 'Do you want to use the john?' she asked.

Gratefully I nodded (I was again too thirsty to speak). She thrust me into a small bathroom off the hall, leaving the door open, and roughly pulled my pants down before I could do it myself. I sat, and she remained standing over me by the open door. I looked up at her, chilled by her expression of disdain and impatience. I was at first unable to let go and feared that she would force me up before I could relieve myself. But at last I succeeded, and even managed to pull up my slacks before she could do it for me. We continued round the corner to what seemed to be a conventional kitchen with an old-fashioned stove and several small tables in the centre. The room was smaller than our cell, and the tables close together. The nurse deposited me at one of the tables and grabbed a plate full of food from the stove. It was an ample and appetizing meal, including a large chicken leg with thigh, a baked potato, and some vegetables. Grateful tears welled in my eyes, for I was hungry, and the food looked good. I was even able to enjoy this fleeting pleasure in some privacy, because the nurses were occupied in placing the other inmates at their seats.

Then I realized that I had no utensils for my meal, and I tried to get the attention of one of the nurses. I could not call to her, for they had not yet given me any water for my dry mouth. When she saw me, I gestured and managed to whisper 'knife and fork, some water please'. In response she tossed me a large, serving-size spoon, which I regarded in disbelief. I weakly poked at my chicken and baked potato, but cutting them with the spoon was an impossibility, and my strange physical numbness and shakiness made it difficult even to hold the spoon firmly. As I tried to move my food around I also found that my eyesight was becoming blurred, and I felt a kind of terror at sitting still in this small room with all the other woman and with the three nurses hovering over us like guards.

'I can't eat like this', I complained.
'Everybody else does', was the reply. 'Do you think you are something special?'

I bowed my head in shame and put down the serving spoon. Well, I had always eaten chicken with my hands anyway, so I picked up the leg and bit into it. Then I did the same with the baked potato, breaking the skin with my teeth. When I was about halfway through, the nurse finally slapped a glass of milk in front of my plate. I downed the milk in one gulp. That ended the meal; it was the best I could do.

The evening in this place was the same as the afternoon. After dinner we were all herded back into the cell to sit for another interminable period. Finally it was time for pills and bath and bed, to which the nurses dragged us as they had at dinner. Again I swallowed a fat brown pill. My bath consisted of a damp washcloth rubbed across my face. My bedroom was a small cell off the other end of the hall. The nurses had changed shifts, and my new nurse was a slight woman with dark hair.

Somehow she seemed to know me better than the other nurses had.

'So you're feeling better today, eh Sally?', she asked me brusquely.
'I guess so', I answered cautiously, not recognizing her either.
'My name is Margaret', said the nurse. 'I've been putting you to bed for the last two weeks. This is the first time you've talked to me. It looks like you are getting better now, eh? Maybe you'll be out of this place soon, eh? You be a good girl. Get out of this place soon. It is good that you are talking.'

All the while she was speaking, she was roughly removing my clothes, replacing them with what I recognized as the pale blue silk pyjamas from Bonwit's that my mother had given me for Christmas. But they were badly ripped in several places.

'What happened to my pyjamas?' I asked.
'You have been very difficult these last two weeks', was all that Margaret would say. She guided me to the bed in the tiny cell, and turned to go. 'You be a good girl', she said. 'Get out of this place, eh?' Then she closed the door – and locked it behind her.

West Hill Hospital was an expensive private hospital in the Riverdale section of the Bronx. Dr Pacella, my doctor, owned and operated West Hill as well as Regency Hospital, a smaller facility above his office on fashionable East 61st Street in Manhattan.

Like many other mental institutions at that time, West Hill had a three-level residential programme, each with a bland name such as 'West Cottage' or 'Thompson', but each in effect representing levels of Dantean misery, various degrees of incarceration and forced treatment. At West Hill, for example, the place I was first taken could be called the hell unit.

From the outside, hell appeared to be a small Victorian cottage nestled beside tastefully landscaped grounds. But inside that quaint cottage the patients were locked up all day long in the large cell, or group seclusion room, with its broken TV set and smell of urine. Patients never saw a doctor and were not allowed to communicate with friends or relatives. Many never left that cottage, or left only to be placed in nursing homes. Their only treatment was intentional neglect along with heavy psychiatric drugging. The brown M&M pills that I was given were 1200 mg a day of thorazine. The drugs had caused my physical sluggishness and trembling, as well as my drastic thirst, for in those days there were no pills to counter such side-effects.

The second residential unit, where I next went, also looked like a respectable summer cottage. But this second unit was a kind of purgatory. Here at least hope was extended that I might eventually be transferred to the main building and someday released from the hospital. The doors of this building were locked, and the staff controlled patients with an iron hand – you did as you were told. Mail was censored and sometimes confiscated, but we were allowed weekly visits from our families. Here at least there was a kind of confused communication among patients and staff; in the day room people actually moved around, and there was a TV in working order. Again, patients were restricted to that room for most of the day; we were locked out of our bedrooms and physically dragged back to the TV area if we ventured into the hall.

The main building at the head of the path was a two-storey mansion with spacious rooms and expensive furniture. This unit represented limbo, with a façade of dreamlike normalcy in which well-behaved patients were free to walk around the lovely grounds, at least on days when they were not incapacitated by shock treatments. On those mornings, most patients received a jolt of electricity, and reclined for the rest of the day on one of the *chaises-longues* in the day room. Except for the undead appearance of the patients, this limbo had every appearance of leisurely gentility.

As soon as I was transferred to purgatory my mother appeared in full battle gear: wearing her flowing pink coat and carrying letters that she had written to me in hell that were only now returned to her unopened. I gave her a letter that I had managed to save before it could be confiscated. 'I have been told that this is a "sanitarium"', I wrote. 'It isn't. It is a snake pit worse than can ever be imagined. Here the time goes by very self-consciously. There is no privacy. It is a wonder that people who come here even remain alive (including me).' Mother took this letter home with her, and years later I found it carefully saved among her other papers.

As soon as she saw the actual conditions in purgatory, mother began an unrelenting campaign to have me transferred to limbo. Her advocacy was fuelled by righteous indignation at the censorship and interception of our mail. Once I was in the main building, Dr Pacella wanted to start electroshock treatments immediately, but mother kept fighting and refused to sign the release form needed to administer shock.

Unfortunately, the fighting spirit that I had mustered in my letter to mother was soon squelched. Soon after I had been transferred to purgatory, I saw Dr Pacella for the first time since my admission. Nobody saw him more than once a week, as he only visited the hospital on Saturdays and the rest of the time conducted hospital business from his plush East Side office. My first visit with him was almost as much of a shock as had been my experience in the hell unit. I was eager to discuss with him what had happened to me in my room at Sarah Lawrence, for I still remembered my spiritual insights and innocently believed that understanding what I had experienced was important to my recovery.

But Dr Pacella refused to talk about it, and even refused to listen to what I had to say. 'You were a very sick girl', he said over and over again. 'I thought you were never going to come out of it.' Immediately I visualized the other women in that group cell, most of whom, apparently, never would 'come out of it'.

Dr Pacella went on to describe how catatonic I had been. He said that I was schizophrenic and that nothing that I had ever thought and nothing that happened to me had anything to do with what was now wrong in my brain. His message was that even my curiosity about what had happened to me was sick and dangerous. It was pointless for me to express any opinion whatsoever. What was there to say?

'Do you believe in God?' I asked Dr Pacella, a practising Roman Catholic.
'We don't need to get into that here', he replied. 'That has nothing to do with what we are doing here.'

What were we doing there? I would still like to know. I know that without any spiritual guidance whatsoever and without some acknowledgement of what I then saw as an enormous spiritual loss, I lapsed into an agony of despair worse than the existential hollowness that I had suffered at the college. I sat day after day among blank-faced men and women lined up in their *chaises-longues* around the sides of the sunny glassed-in porch of limbo-land. All of us were deliberately reduced to abject dependence upon a system of sanity that required the maintenance of a strict control on any emotion or mental energy. Recovery was synonymous with the erasure of any individual beliefs or hopes except those standardized by society as represented by Dr Pacella. I myself came to believe that if there was any meaning in the world, it was known only to Dr Pacella and his nurses, and perhaps the rest of the world, but was forever lost to me. I had lost not just my education and my future, but even my soul.

Dr Pacella would not talk with me about anything more profound than my eating and sleeping patterns, and our visits at West Hill never lasted more than ten minutes. Never once was I allowed to describe what had happened in my mind and heart or to express what it meant to me.

I left West Hill in late June, after nearly five months. Mother picked me up and brought me back to her tiny one-bedroom apartment in the Village. As she prepared a tea tray for us, I sat bleakly in the living room, baffled at the strangeness of the outside world. I felt out of place, grotesquely out of place, something like Kafka's cockroach trying to become assimilated into polite society. Physically, I felt wretched. I could not even see properly; although I tilted my head in several different directions the room always seemed to shimmer and blur. An unfamiliar heaviness in my body made me feel that I could not even cope with the motions required to get up and go to the bathroom. Whatever was I going to do with myself? Sarah Lawrence refused to take me back; they were now demanding that I clear my belongings out of my old room with no further delay. I could not face going there, I was so ashamed. I could not bear the thought of encountering my old friends. I was now a cockroach, and my friends were studying for their bachelor's degree. What was I going to do with myself? I could not even read now, much less go back to school, even if they would take me. I could not sit and tremble like an insect all day in a cosy apartment. Although I felt like a cockroach, I could not even take refuge in the cracks in the walls.

I was at that time still under a heavy dose of thorazine. Had I been told that the sluggishness and trembling, and the difficulty in reading, were side-effects of the medication I was taking, I might not have panicked as I did. But these effects had never been explained to me, and what had been tolerable in the confinement of the hospital became unbearable in the real world. As far as I knew, these agonies were signs of my own weakness and continuing illness, and they made me hate myself.

When mother appeared with the tea tray and cheerfully began her ritual of pouring and stirring, I just slumped in my chair and began to cry. I could not explain; I did not even bother to cover my contorted face. 'I can't do it', was all I could say. 'Take me back.'

The last six weeks of my first institutionalization were spent in Regency Hospital, a ward of single rooms that occupied the floor above Dr Pacella's office on 61st Street. Patients were not encouraged to 'fraternize' with each other, so although I spent a good amount of time padding up and down the ward in my robe and slippers, I seldom met or talked with any of the other patients. As I passed by their rooms, I glimpsed solitary figures lying on their beds watching TV or sitting wistfully by windows that opened to views of brick walls or street lights. The other patients seldom looked back at me.

My father, who had cheerfully paid the bills during my months of confinement, stepped up his stream of get-well cards to me. Because I was now allowed out of the unit for brief trips, my stepmother flew to New York and tried to cheer me up by taking me to Bloomingdales. At about that time the thorazine was also reduced, and my head began to clear. Instead of worrying about the fog in my head, I now felt more like myself. Still too vulnerable to venture into the outside world alone, I began to take a new interest in outside events through the TV set. I particularly enjoyed watching game shows such as Password and Concentration. In the days before screaming audiences, these shows actually provided a little mental exercise as well as entertainment. I was encouraged that my brain still functioned.

Shortly after I entered the Regency, Dr Pacella persuaded mother to sign a release for insulin shock treatments. I do not know how he accomplished this; certainly he neglected to tell her that the coma caused by insulin is even more dangerous than the convulsions produced by electricity.

I myself did not fully appreciate what was being done to me. On a treatment day, several nurses entered my room in the morning while I was watching my TV shows. They injected me with insulin, and within seconds I dropped into a deep coma. I did not awaken until late afternoon, when another gaggle of nurses surrounded me and poured orange juice down my throat. The nurses had to spend several minutes prodding me, even though I was trying as hard as I could to wake up. It was very confusing. After a treatment, I could not understand who all these people were, where I was, and what time of day it was. For the remainder of the afternoon and evening on I could only lie limply on my bed, starring at the TV and wondering in a dazed way what was going on.

After six weeks of insulin coma treatment, Dr Pacella again deemed that I was ready to go out into the world. It is true that I was no longer wrapped up in despair and worry. I scarcely remembered who I was, and if reminded that I had been attending college or that I had had any friends, I regarded the information as something out of long-past history. As for any personal ambitions or spiritual needs, I did not think of these things at all. Mother had told me that she had arranged for us to share with her friend Gerry a summer cottage on a lake, and that she was enquiring about a secretarial school for me to attend in the fall. Fine. I was happy to have all the decisions made for me.

I was mildly pleased when my old suitemate Carol came to visit, bearing a small bouquet of chrysanthemums. I smiled at her blankly and let her do all the talking. She talked about her painting and some of our mutual friends. I did not even consider mentioning my crack-up, of finally reviewing my spiritual drama with someone who had witnessed it first hand. All of that was long ago. I did not care.

The Wounded Prophet

Moses said to the Lord, 'O Lord, I have never been eloquent, neither in the past nor since you have spoken to your servant. I am slow of speech and tongue'. (Exodus 4:10)

Moses stuttered. His disability remained even after he had been to the mountain top and returned with the authority to lead his people. It is why his brother Aaron had to act as his spokesperson. Moses never recovered.

Recovery is the latest buzz word in the mental health field. For the last year or so, I have been labelled 'recovered from mental illness'. I acquired this label when the Office of Mental Health in New York State invited me to participate in their Recovery Dialogues. I was one of a select group of consumer/survivors chosen to discuss the concept of recovery with a group of psychiatrists. These dialogues are ongoing, and they have been very interesting. We have covered a wide range of topics, from complaints about mental health treatment more damaging than healing; to consumer participation in the education of psychiatrists; to personal descriptions of madness; to coping techniques and the management of symptoms.

What the discussions have failed to address, however, is the nature of mental illness itself. Several of us in the 'recovered' category have described our extreme mental states in the hope that these might inspire examination of what really happens in the mind, as well as the body, of the person labelled mentally ill. If we are recovered, what is it that we have recovered from? If we are well now and were sick before, what is it that we have recovered to? For some reason this discussion never gets off the ground. The psychiatrists in our dialogue become visibly uneasy when the subject arises, and they divert the discussion to a less threatening line of thought. 'Coping mechanisms' are just such a diversion, an attempt to regard the depth of madness as something that can be simply 'coped' with.

It only makes sense that, if we are 'ill', then this illness must have an objective marker. Diabetes, for example, is identified by a blood test that reveals a deficiency of insulin. AIDS is identified by a virus in the blood-stream. Cancer is identified by a tumorous growth visible on X-rays. But mental illness has as yet no objective marker. Although it is widely specu-lated that brain chemistry is the culprit, there is no laboratory test that will reveal the biochemical nature of our illness, or even whether or not we are ill at all. Genetic markers for manic depression have been announced, and then found to be mistaken. The truth is that the current state of the art for psychiatric diagnosis is based solely on the subjective observation of external behaviour – not a very objective marker for a process that is internal.

Those of us who have had the experience called 'mental illness' know in our hearts that something profound is missing in these diagnoses. They do not take into account what we have actually endured. Even if the 'bad' chemical or the 'defective' gene is someday found, madness has its own reality that demands attention. There is something compelling about the experience of an altered state, something that Ed Podvoll calls *The Seduction of Madness* (Podvoll, 1990). What is compelling about madness is the tantalizing hint that it holds the secrets of consciousness, of healing and of spiritual power. It is madness that brings the mind to our atten-tion, that makes us remember that mind is inseparable from spirit, that it is consciousness that makes us human. A great Buddhist lama once wrote:

> Spirituality, self-existing, radiant,
> In which there is no memory to upset you
> Cannot be called a thing. (Tilopa, 1963)

For me, becoming 'mentally ill' was always a spiritual crisis, and finding a spiritual model of recovery was a question of life or death. My search began over 30 years ago, when I took time off from college studies to shut myself in my room alone to find God and the meaning of life. For a week or so, I listened to music, entertained myself with mental images, and had spiritual revelations. I experienced many unusual perceptions and bodily changes similar to ones that occur with drugs such as LSD. All of this climaxed with a vision of the oneness and interdependence of everything in the universe – the sort of thing that sounds foolish when put into words, but is profoundly true for those who experience it.

But my extreme mental state did not wear off the way drugs eventually do. After a while my mood turned ugly and destructive – like a 'bad trip' that would not end. I struck the school nurse, breaking her arm, and I plunged into a hell of darkness and despair. When I did not eat or sleep or talk to my friends, the college called an ambulance to pick me up. The attendants gave me a shot of thorazine, put me into a strait-jacket, and carried me off. At the mental hospital I was diagnosed with schizophrenia, locked in seclusion for several weeks, and drugged with 1200 mg a day of thorazine. Later the doctor told me that my entire experience with spiritual ecstasy and darkness was sick and irrational, and had no meaning whatsoever. Shamed, I stayed in the hospital for five months, and by the time I got out I was a sadly different person from the one who had seen God just a few months before. I was defeated. I considered myself a complete and utter failure for the rest of my life. God was gone.

I was not allowed to return to college, and most of the people who had been my friends would no longer talk to me. I felt so weak and degraded that I could not work, and I enrolled in secretarial school only because my mother insisted. After a year I was well enough to get married and find a job. I did well on the job, but after six months I suddenly cracked up again and wound up back in hospital. Since then I have been hospitalized over 18 times, once for as long as two years.

I have been given just about every psychiatric drug in the medical armoury: major tranquillizers, minor tranquillizers, antidepressants, mood elevators, sleeping pills, lithium, and Prozac. I have spent more days in seclusion rooms than I can count, and I have been tied down in five-point restraints. I have received both insulin shock and electric shock. Few of these 'treatments' helped me at all, and most of them damaged me badly. They left me debilitated and desperate. One might wonder why am I still standing at all. I certainly owe no thanks to the mental health system. The faith in my inner experience always returned to strengthen me; it is only this spiritual outlook that enabled me to go on.

As a child I had loved the silent time before the liturgy began at church. I would kneel on the prayer bench for a long time, absorbed in silence. In high school, without giving a name to what I did, I often sat alone in my room or outside in the mountains or woods, and I learned to trust the peace and confidence that this brought. Oddly enough, I did not realize how precious this was, for at the time it was simply a part of who I was and what I liked to do. Spirituality is like that – it is so close to you that it may not seem very important. Because I had faith in my mind, and trusted it, I never lost touch with fundamental reality, even when later I became depressed or manic or fearful. Whether my thoughts became threatening or blissful, I knew that behind them all was spiritual stillness. I knew that although my emotions may arise from brain chemicals, or may themselves trigger chemical changes, the form my emotions take and the meaning I give them are my responsibility.

Even after the horrible treatment that I received in every single one of the mental hospitals, secretly I cherished the spiritual vision of my altered states. That could not be erased, because it was real. Even when depression and despair followed a manic episode, my vision of truth prevailed over the sorry platitudes and euphemisms offered as help by friends and therapists. Those lies were never real in the way that my vision was. Nevertheless, for 15 years I lived a lie. I tried to regard my spiritual experiences as symptoms of illness, and dutifully kept my life safe and dull and meaningless. It never worked. Inevitably my mind would go its own way, and I would once again wind up in a mental institution.

My healing did not begin until 1978, fifteen years after my first hospitalization. I began to study and practise Buddhism, where I found a comprehensive psychology of the mind and specific methods to overcome confusion and suffering. I found descriptions of mental states identical to those I had experienced when 'mentally ill'. Most of all, I found psychology presented as part of a spiritual process, a psychology of the heart (Govinda, 1969; Freemantle and Trungpa, 1975; Trungpa, 1972). Finally I could admit openly that my experiences were, and always had been, a spiritual journey – not sick, shameful, or evil. I was already a worthwhile person, right from the start, and there was a way to work with my own mind to transform fearful mental states to peaceful ones.

Of course nothing is as simple as that. I found at first that sitting on a meditation cushion in Buddhist fashion was very difficult to do when my mind was disturbed. I could not keep up with the people who meditated for hours at a time at the centres I attended. Finally I spoke about this to a Tibetan lama in Woodstock, New York, and I honestly admitted my diagnosis of mental illness. With trepidation, I confessed my conviction that I gained precious spiritual insights from my experiences. Unlike

Western friends and therapists, he did not try to convince me that my spiritual concerns were trivial and just another symptom of mental illness. He took what I said seriously, and his advice was that I bring my understanding into the community, and use it to help others.

That is how I began working as a peer advocate and counsellor. After my talk with the lama, I first volunteered for the Red Cross in Portland, Maine, and worked on their disaster team. Then I found a small group of psychiatric survivors and organized the Portland Coalition for the Psychiatrically Labelled. Little by little I learned how to give peer support to other people, and how to advocate for them within the mental health system. The more I did this work, the more confidence I gained in myself. For the first time since college, I started to feel like a real person, somebody worthy of respect. Not only that, I began to receive respect, not just from other ex-patients, but also from people in the community.

As I gained in confidence and in the practice of compassion, I found it easier to practise the mental disciplines I had been taught. I began doing meditation for 20 minutes a day, and I also went back to church and joined the choir, for I have always enjoyed singing. Still, I kept 'going off the deep end' and had to be rehospitalized almost on a yearly basis. Weary of battling these psychotic episodes, and overstressed by my work, in 1988 I returned to Woodstock and took an apartment near the Tibetan monastery. I hoped that spiritual practice would help me clear away anger and fear, the emotions that caused my mental states to get out of control. My teacher, Khenpo Karthar Rinpoche, gave me individual instructions. I was assigned the practice of the Green Tara Sadhana, a chanting meditation in praise of Tara, a female deity of compassion and wisdom (Willson, 1986). For two years, I practised intensively at KTD Monastery, and I heard oral teachings from many high Tibetan lamas. Hearing the teachings confirmed to me that my spiritual interpretation of manic experiences was valid, and my insights were genuine.

After this period, I again ventured out into the world. I volunteered on a local 24-hour community hotline, and joined peer support groups in two nearby towns. Within a couple of years I organized the support groups into a non-profit corporation called PEOPLe: Projects to Empower and Organize the Psychiatrically Labelled. Modelled after the Portland Coalition, PEOPLe became a force for advocacy and a resource for support throughout the Hudson Valley in New York.

It has now been eight years since I have been committed to a mental institution. Although I cannot claim stability in my life, much less enlightenment, my anger and fear are greatly reduced, and my impulses no longer drive me over the edge into madness. More than ever, I am convinced that this recovery, if you can call it that, is the result of my spiritual practice. The faith that I learned long ago from silent prayer made it easier for me to understand my mental states without fear. The Green Tara Sadhana, a kind of yoga, allowed me to stabilize my mental state by integrating mind and body. The help that I have given other people taught me compassion.

But I must also give a certain amount of credit to my madness itself. When I came to study at the monastery and listened to the high lamas, I compared what I heard with what I had experienced. It all fitted together. Everything that the lamas taught about the nature of the mind coincided with what I had already learned within my altered states of consciousness. From the lamas I learned how very important it is that we respect our consciousness, in all its dimensions. It is a house of many mansions.

The questions remain. If mental illness is a disease of the mind, what is the nature of the mind? If altered states have value, what is there to recover from? What is our model of wellness? Is it true, as some say, that spiritual realization is the highest aspiration of the human race? If it is, should not that be our model of wellness? How do we recover to that state of wellness? Is recovery for a mental patient something different from the wellness of any other person?

Why do people in mania consistently experience an urgent call to save the world, and call themselves messiah or saviour? Is this merely grandiose, or do such people truly hear a call to help others?

We know that people called schizophrenic hear voices. But why do they listen to them? Why in this culture are some forms of mental illness so excruciatingly painful and so interminable? Is illness the reason, or is there a tragic misunderstanding of global proportions? Who is ill – is it the visionary or is it the society itself?

We now know that mental illness appears in a very high proportion of creative artists and world leaders. Some of those who have achieved greatness in spite of – or even because of – mental affliction are the artist Vincent Van Gogh, poet Robert Lowell, and President Abraham Lincoln. Is this a fluke, or is there actually an indispensable link between madness and creativity?

For centuries, ever since human beings emerged as distinct from apes in the chain of evolution, people have experienced extreme mental states. In most societies, altered states of mind have held a place of respect, and have served to give spiritual meaning to the culture. In indigenous cultures, for example, the shamanistic tradition involves an individual's journey through his or her own mind. This journey is typically painful and even turbulent, but, because the people who experience it are guided through it by spiritual elders and the community itself, they emerge from their ordeal with new-found wisdom and the power to heal.

Eastern peoples believe that mental disturbance is a question of both body and soul. Although emotions come from the brain, the mind is located in the heart, not the head. Mind and heart are synonymous. Thus the brain is part of the body, but the mind is part of the spirit. In the ancient Hindu scripture, the Bhagavad-Gita, called the 'Song of God', it says: 'One must elevate oneself by one's own mind, not degrade oneself. The mind is the friend of the human soul, and its enemy as well' (Murray and Murray, 1980). In ancient Tibetan medicine, madness was considered the easiest of all maladies to cure, and it was treated with the use of herbs, diet and spiritual practices (Clifford, 1984). Buddhism, like other contemplative traditions, uses the discipline of meditation to open up dimensions of extra-ordinary mental states that lead to spiritual wellness.

Even the Judeo-Christian religions are founded upon the inner experience of the heart. When Moses went up to the mountain, he experienced an altered state of mind. He had a vision – you might say hallucination – of a burning bush, and a face-to-face encounter with something for which he had no name, and which terrified him.

There the angel of the Lord appeared to him in flames of fire from within a bush. Moses saw that though the bush was on fire it did not burn up. So Moses thought, I will go over and see this strange sight – why the bush does not burn up. When the Lord saw that he had gone over to look, God called to him from within the bush, 'Moses, Moses!' And Moses said, 'Here I am'.

Yahweh told Moses that he was being sent to bring the Israelites out of Egypt. Moses said to Yahweh, 'Suppose I go to the Israelites and say to them, "The God of your fathers has sent me to you", and they ask me, "What is His name?". Then what shall I tell them?' God said to Moses, 'I am that I am. This is what you are to say to the Israelites: I AM has sent me to you.' (Exodus 3:2–14)

It was this experience that made Moses a prophet. Later, of course, he received the Ten Commandments and brought the stone tablets to his people. But that was later. The experience that enabled Moses to lead his people to the promised land was an altered state of consciousness. And many of us who have been labelled mentally ill know first hand what that altered state is like.

We know what the 'I am' is. If we are Buddhists we know what 'suchness' is. If we are shamans, we know who we are.

Until recent times, altered states of the kind I have described were an integral – and integrated – part of human experience. Among the ways they were incorporated into society were the shamanistic/healing way, the contemplative/teaching way, and the prophetic/leadership way. It is only recently that altered states have been medicalized and stigmatized. It is only recently that powerful drugs have been used to suppress the altered states that once produced our prophets and our saints.

Not surprisingly, it is also recently that society has fallen into a spiritual crisis of unprecedented proportions. In case you had not noticed, we no longer have any shamans or prophets. There may be those who go by those names, but somehow the mental experience that shapes such people is missing. This lack is sorely felt. We are lost now, lost on a global scale. Our world has lost its meaning, and our religions have lost their authority.

Not surprisingly, millions of people today are seeking to reach an altered state in the only way that they know how: through the use of mind-altering drugs. We may try with all our might to get rid of the drugs, but as long as we are human, we will not get rid of the need for altered states.

Buddhism identifies two components of spiritual realization: wisdom and compassion. It prescribes meditation to attain mental clarity and good works to learn compassion. The intimate experience of mind through meditation opens the heart to compassion. Similarly, the good that we do for ourselves and others opens our minds to wisdom. The Bhagavad-Gita says, 'One whose mind is controlled and who strives by right means is assured of success' (Murray and Murray, 1980). And Jesus was talking about the same two activities when he named the two great commandments (Matthew 22:37–39). The first is to 'love the Lord your God with all your heart and with all your soul and with all your mind'. This corresponds to wisdom. The second great commandment is to 'love your neighbour as yourself' – and this is the same as compassion.

For me, Dharma practice was healing, for I found that the two Buddhist aspects of enlightenment – wisdom and compassion – are prescriptions for mental wellness in general. By following them, I achieved what others have called 'recovery'. But clarity and love are not restricted to Eastern religions, and we need not turn to esoteric practices to find a cure for mental suffering. We do, however, need to re-examine mental health treatment from the perspective of mental states – in other words consciousness. I believe that any meaningful treatment for mental illness must have a spiritual basis.

Any model of healing the mind must begin by acknowledging the spiritual properties inherent in altered states. It will include a human exchange between client and provider, one in which the client can share and even transmit what he or she has learned. People who have experienced madness have something to give back to the world. It is no coincidence that we are likely to be sensitive thinkers, talented in the arts, and understanding of others. Many of us have seen the 'I am', have understood the 'suchness' of phenomena, and want to help others.

Mental health professionals need to study the dimensions of consciousness, and to learn to practise compassion and wisdom themselves. These inner disciplines can and should be taught to anyone entering the field of mental health. Persons suffering from mental confusion may need medical technology, and even drugs, to help them 'cope'. But any good psychiatrist, psychologist, or mental health worker must first be a decent human being – and certified as such!

When we talk about finding a 'cure' for mental illness, it is important to expand the definition of sanity to include clarity and compassion that can coexist within so-called 'symptoms'. Health, or sanity, can be achieved even within an affliction or disability. As examples, both Franklin Delano Roosevelt and Helen Keller were severely physically disabled, yet one became the leader and the other the teacher of millions of people. In my case, the healing process and my successful work as a peer advocate started while I was still suffering periodic breakdowns, and continued for some time while I was still going in and out of hospital.

Few of us who have been psychiatrically labelled would claim to have recovered to the point where we no longer experience our manic energy, our depression, our voices, or even our confusion. It is embarrassing, but I must admit that for the last six months I have been quite depressed myself. I do not think I will ever again get so out of control that I will have to be hospitalized. But even if that should happen, I will not lose faith in my experience and my journey. I take comfort in another lesson that I learned from the Tibetan lamas. These holy people, and holy people I have met in other traditions, are remarkable for their very humanness. They have quirks and foibles and frailties, but these in no way contradict their spiritual realization.

Often ex-patients and patients within the community are expected to endure lives like those we see all around us. Everywhere these days we see people living lives of quiet desperation – lives, as Kierkegaard noted, of 'indifference, so remote from the good that they are almost too spiritless to be called sin, yes almost too spiritless to be called despair' (Kierkegaard, 1954). We who have experienced mental illness have all learned the same thing, whether our extreme mental states were inspiring or frightening. We know that we have reached the bare bones of spirit and of what it means to be human. Whatever our suffering, we know that we do not want to become automatons, or to wear the false façade that others adopt.

Whether we have had revelations or have hit rock bottom, most of us have also suffered from the ignorance of those who fear to look at what we have seen, who always try to change the subject. Although we have been broken, we have tasted the marrow of reality. There is something to be learned here about the mystery of living itself, something important both to those who have suffered and those who seek to help us. We must teach each other.

We must teach each other, knowing that it is often the wounded healer, or the wounded prophet, who is most able to help others. The stigma that we bear need not be a mark of shame. Instead, like Jacob after he wrestled with the angel, we can wear our disability as a badge of honour. In Jacob's first altered state, he received a wound that stayed with him for the rest of his life:

> That night, after Jacob had sent his family across the stream, he sent over all his possessions. So [he] was left alone, and a man wrestled with him until daybreak. When the man saw that he could not overpower him, he touched the socket of Jacob's hip so that his hip was wrenched as he wrestled with the man. Then the man said, 'let me go, for it is daybreak'. But Jacob replied, 'I will not let you go unless you bless me'. The man asked him, 'What is your name?'. 'Jacob', he answered. Then the man said, 'Your name will no longer be Jacob, but Israel, because you have struggled with God and with men and overcome'. (Genesis 32:22–28)

Jacob named the place of his struggle Peniel, which means 'face of God'. I, too, have seen God face to face, and I want to remember my Peniel. I really do not want to be called recovered. From the experience of madness I received a wound that changed my life. It enabled me to help others and to know myself. I am proud that I have struggled with God and with the mental health system.

I have not recovered. I have overcome.

References

Clifford T (1984) Tibetan Buddhist Medicine and Psychiatry. The Diamond Healing. York Beach, ME: Samuel Weiser.

Freemantle F, Chogyam Trungpa (1975) The Tibetan Book of the Dead. The Great Liberation Through Hearing in the Bardo. Boulder, CO and London, UK: Shambhala.

Govinda Lama Anagarika (1969) Foundations of Tibetan Mysticism. New York: Samuel Weiser.

Holy Bible, New International Version (n.d.) Grand Rapids, MI: Zondervan Bible Publishers.

Kierkegaard S (1954) Appendix to The Sickness Unto Death. Garden City, NY: Doubleday Anchor, p 232.

Murray K, Murray C (1980) Illuminations from the Bhagavad-Gita. New York: Harper & Row.

Podvoll EM (1990) The Seduction of Madness. Revolutionary Insights into the World of Psychosis and a Compassionate Approach to Recovery at Home. New York: HarperCollins.

Tilopa (1963) Song of Oral Instructions. The Life and Teaching of Naropa. Translated by Herbert V Guenther. New York: Oxford University Press, p 95.

Trungpa Chogyam (1972) Mudra. Berkeley: Shambhala.

Willson M (1986) In Praise of Tara. Songs to the Saviouress. London: Wisdom Publications.

Chapter 3
The Other World

Jan Holloway

Editorial

One of the enduring myths of mental health care is that professionals have some kind of immunity to mental illness of any kind. Increasingly, we recognize that staff are prone to 'stress' and more recently to 'burnout'. The pressures of crazy systems and abusive management practices often result in demoralized staff, some of whom become clinically depressed. These forms of mental distress are sometimes accepted as 'reasonable' responses to wholly unreasonable work or living conditions. When our colleagues experience more 'serious mental illness', the fear, avoidance and general retreat from contact of colleagues – even friends – adds a singular insult to the original injury. Jan Holloway's story is a remarkable tale of just such an experience, and of her survival and rebirth. The difficulty for anyone in rising from the ashes of their experience of madness cannot be exaggerated. Where the person is a senior health care professional, the act of reclaiming both personal and professional identities demands not only courage but also perseverance. Jan Holloway appears to have had an adequate supply of both.

For new mental health care staff who have also themselves been service users, an important component of induction and training packages appears to be the opportunity to reflect, preferably within a group of people in like situations, on the transition from being service user to service provider. The opportunity to think through the implications of self-disclosure, both within the staff team and in relation to patients in their care, proves to be similarly important. Jan addresses herself, through her narrative, to both of these issues, not only offering a powerful account of her own struggle, but providing a valuable training resource which clinicians will use increasingly as a springboard for their own professional development.

*　*　*　*　*

Prologue[4]

The voice was getting louder as I walked into the psychiatric day centre.

'Kill or be killed', it was telling me. *'Kill or be killed.'*

There were a few people around who smiled at me and I managed to say hello as I walked up the stairs, hoping no one would stop me to talk. I just wanted to sit on my own and have a cigarette. But upstairs ten staff were sitting around a table waiting for me. I looked around the faces, wondering what they knew.

'Kill or be killed.'

I managed to say good morning, pulled up a chair and rummaged in my bag for my tobacco. I could feel the cells of my body moving around. Someone was moving them. Someone was moving the cells around in my brain, controlling my thoughts. It was not safe to speak. I pulled out my tobacco, checking for the large penknife that lay in the bottom of my bag. It was reassuring.

'Kill or be killed.'

Someone else was talking but I could not concentrate on what they were saying. I lit my cigarette and looked up.

'What do you think, Jan?'
'Kill or be killed.'

Ten faces were waiting expectantly. What did they know? It was not safe to speak but I knew I would have to. I had to say something because I was the manager of the day centre.

Part 1: Professional

At the start of 1991 I was 33 years old and I had been qualified as an occupational therapist for 11 years. I came from a working-class family, the elder of two sisters, and had been epileptic since the age of 18. Despite this I had worked consistently in a variety of rewarding jobs culminating in my first managerial position as team leader of The Grange Day Centre, one of the first projects for the rehabilitation of long-stay psychiatric patients. I had always felt my greatest skills lay in the mental health field

---

[4] Acknowledgement. I should like to record my debt to Sally Cameron for the help she gave me with this chapter, particularly for the skilled and sensitive way she put my thoughts and experiences, and our conversations about them, in order. Sadly, Sally died on 10 June 1996 and this was her last piece of writing. I believe this is a fitting memory of her abilities as a writer and her qualities as a dear friend.

and, although it was sometimes a struggle, I enjoyed my work immensely. At home I lived happily with Paul, my partner of 14 years.

I had experienced only one period of what could be called mental disease, but this was many years before, when I was 18 and had become quite depressed. However, this depression was short lived and easily explainable as a reaction to my recent diagnosis of epilepsy coupled with the pressure of school exams. In 1991 I did not consider myself to be mentally ill. I *worked* with the mentally ill. This is not to say, of course, that I was always happy. Who is? I still had a lot of unresolved feelings around being epileptic and I had been seeing a psychotherapist for five years, which I found useful. Many of my colleagues were also in therapy and I felt it could only benefit my work and increase my understanding of the role of 'patient'.

Increasingly, however, I had begun to feel that my problems were not so much centred on my epilepsy as on my close relationships. Surprising, it seemed, as I had always had lots of friends and a loving and stable relationship with Paul. But gradually I began to feel that the people I was closest to, Paul, my close friends and my psychotherapist, were beginning to have too much power over me. I think I first became fully aware of the problem when I went off on holiday with three of my closest friends, Trini, Janice and Jaina, to a beautiful cottage in Wales. It should have been an idyllic time, perfect surroundings with people whom I loved and who loved me, but the reality soon became a nightmare. I felt overwhelmed, overtaken, without boundaries, and very soon I found myself searching for ways of being alone. It was not hard. In such beautiful countryside it was not at all unusual to want to go off for walks on my own, slip outside alone to watch the sunset. No one realized what was going on, and why should they have? No one could possibly have conceived that I was convinced they were trying to control my thoughts.

This is not an easy idea to grasp because, of course, it defies the logic of the world, and so at this point it is useful to imagine another world, my *other world*, where the rules are very different. In this other world the cells of my brain are tangible to others. They can be moved around, they can be changed, and so my thoughts become vulnerable. People can *know* my thoughts; they can remove them or they can insert thoughts of their own. This kind of power is pretty scary. Fortunately, however, I knew what to do. I had spent 11 years reading psychiatric textbooks and working with people who were psychotic. I asked my GP to refer me to a psychiatrist.

I actually saw two psychiatrists. My GP referred me to a psychiatrist at Goodmayes Hospital and my psychotherapist referred me to a psychiatrist at The Westminster Pastoral Foundation. Both told me that there was nothing wrong with me. The Goodmayes psychiatrist said that if I knew I was psychotic then I obviously had insight and therefore could not possibly be psychotic.

'Are you going to work?', he asked me. 'Are you cooking for your boyfriend?'
I said I was.
'Then there is not much wrong with you', he said. 'I can give you some anti-depressants, but don't take them all at once or I'll get into trouble!'

The psychiatrist at the WPF told me not to worry so much about things. He said my problem existed just because of the type of people I worked with.

I did not feel that I had been helped. So I put a penknife in my bag and carried it around at all times, just to be on the safe side.

I was now consistently in a dilemma. On the one hand I felt scared and vulnerable and I wanted very much to be close to people. But at the same time the people I wanted to be close to were becoming increasingly threatening. Meanwhile my therapy was deteriorating rapidly. One day I was sitting talking to my therapist and had the sudden sensation of my brain cells moving. I was convinced it was my therapist controlling my thoughts and I knew that she was going to make me throw myself out of the window. The next time I saw her she said, carefully, 'I think we need to have a break'.

I was not surprised. I knew that I was not fully benefiting from therapy but I thought that perhaps if I could get some anti-psychotic medication to control the bizarre thoughts then I would be able to make more use of therapy.

'For how long will the break be?', I asked tentatively.
'Until you get better', said my therapist.
'Okay', I said. 'When will it start?'
'Now', replied my therapist. 'This is the last session.'

It was an abrupt end to five years. I felt as if I had been thrown into outer space. I floated out of the room. I never saw her again.

Two days later I heard the voice for the first time. It was my therapist's voice. I was sitting at work writing a report and drinking a can of coke.

'She's drinking a can of coke', said the voice.
I immediately reached for my tobacco.
'She's going to roll a cigarette', said the voice.

Thereafter the voice commented on my actions and my thoughts, talking about me in the third person to someone else whom I could not hear. It was like listening to one side of a telephone conversation. Always the same voice, always about me. It made it very hard to concentrate. At work I told no one, but at the same time I was convinced that everyone knew. I did not trust anyone. I knew, as a mental health professional, what the treatment would be if I told everything – without a doubt admission to hospital. I knew that I needed some anti-psychotic medication but I did not know how I was going to get this without ending up in hospital. Paul was worried about me. I no longer wanted to go out in the evenings but I could not tell him why. I sat at home on my own, putting the headphones on my ears and turning the music up loud to drown out the voice. It did not work. The voice just got louder, and now it was not only echoing and commenting, it was offering opinions too.

There was quite a bit of disagreement at work at this time about whether or not to move one of our clients out of hospital and into the residential unit. One staff member, particularly, was berating me for my caution, as I had said that this client, who had a history of arson, would not be safe at The Grange.

'You're not giving her a chance', said the worker.
'*She's useless at her job*', said the voice.
'You're just protecting your own neck', said the worker.
'*She's only pretending to be a manager*', said the voice.

I backed down. Although I knew that the client was expressing increasing, if covert, alarm at the prospect of leaving hospital, I also knew that I was going mad. How could my judgement be correct? Considering the state I was in I had no right to make decisions about other peoples' lives. The worker went off victoriously to tell the client she could move into The Grange. The next day the client set fire to her hospital ward and was admitted to Broadmoor. I knew then, without a shadow of a doubt, that I was no longer managing effectively.

I tried to talk to my line manager but I was still very wary of saying too much. He knew that I had become a bit unstuck in psychotherapy and had sought psychiatric help.

'That proves to me that therapy's no good', he said.

I said little more. I did not want to panic him. Although I was convinced that everyone knew what was going on the reality of the situation was that no one suspected a thing. Some of my colleagues have told me since that I seemed no different, and appeared to be managing well. Considering how fragmented I was, this is quite frightening. I was hearing the voice constantly.

'She's going to kill or be killed. Kill or be killed.'

I was feeling threatened by everyone, and I was carrying a knife which I believed that I might have to use in order to protect myself.

No one noticed.

It was only a week and a half since my last therapy session and things had become unbearable. On the Friday night I told Paul again that I did not want to go out. The voice had become louder, more intense. Its tone was nastier.

'She's going to kill or be killed.'

I was on my own in the house and I knew I was dangerous. I was in the other world, and in the other world there were only two awful options. Either I would kill someone or I would die. I had to protect Paul; I had to protect everyone I cared about. So I decided to kill myself.

The plan seemed pretty efficient. I would take an overdose of phenytoin, my epilepsy medication for which the *British National Formulary* stated there was no antidote. It could therefore look like an accident and so my life insurance and mortgage insurance would not be affected, thus leaving no debt for Paul. I drank a little brandy to relax me and make it easier to swallow all the pills, and I took some maxolon to stop me vomiting them up. My plan had been to walk out on to Wanstead Flats, an isolated area where I knew I would not be found until well and truly dead, but almost immediately I started throwing up violently, and that was how Paul found me when he got home.

I was pretty sure that I had vomited up all the tablets and I was reluctant to go to hospital, but Paul insisted that I went to the GP the following morning. I did not sleep that night and in the morning I arrived at the surgery feeling very fragile and scared. I knew that I wanted to tell her everything but I also knew what that telling would mean. I still hoped that I could just get a prescription – some tranquillizers, chlorpromazine or something, that would control my psychotic symptoms. I still *knew* that they were symptoms, and I knew that there were very specific drugs which could make me feel better. I told her quite a bit. I did not tell her about the voice, or about the knife, but it was enough.

'Do you want to go to hospital?', she asked me.

I did not.

'Is there an alternative?', I asked.
'I don't think so', she replied.
'What do you think?', I asked.
'I think it will be safer for you and other people', she told me.
'Is there any choice?', I asked.
'No, not really', she said. 'If you refuse there won't be a choice.'

So there it was. My internal *other world* was now public and I was deemed a danger to the public at large. I was sectionable. I had left the world of mental health professionals and joined that of the mentally ill patient. It seemed best to go quietly.

Part 2: Patient

The GP began to talk briskly. I was to go to casualty at Newham General Hospital to check my phenytoin levels, and then on to Goodmayes where she would arrange a bed by phone. She dialled the number of Goodmayes and then handed me the receiver.

'Hold the phone a moment', she told me. 'I've just got to water my plants.'

I held the telephone to my ear and watched her climb on a chair with her watering can. In the course of my work I had telephoned psychiatric hospitals many times but this was not quite what I had expected.

'Er – what shall I say?', I asked.
('Hello, I'm a mad bastard – can I come in?')
She looked around casually.
'Oh, just tell them to hold for a minute.'

I listened to the ringing tone and watched her watering the plants. Thankfully there was no reply until she had stepped down, replaced the watering can and taken the phone from me. Yes, there was a bed.

I went back home where Paul was waiting for me, having taken the day off work. I packed a bag. We stopped at the tobacconist's where I bought three packets of Gauloise tobacco, and then went on to Newham General where I was seen quickly. It seemed surprising that everyone was so nice to me. Paul came with me in the ambulance to Goodmayes and seemed worried when we walked into the reception area and saw patients lying on the floor. But I knew the score. I explained to him that the patients were not allowed to sleep in their beds during the day and so they would sleep anywhere they could, drugged up as they were. On the ward, waiting to see the doctor, I was still hoping that I would only be there for a couple of days, perhaps get a good dose of tranquillizers and then be able to go home. Looking around at the other patients I felt nervous. Supposing they realized who I was, what I did for a living? Would they hate me? A spy in the camp? Then a young female patient came up to me, Sybil. She was friendly, energetic, warm. Her clinical description could have been manic. She was also training as a psychiatric nurse, five months away from qualifying when she had had a breakdown. It was reassuring.

After a long wait I saw the doctor and he suggested chlorpromazine, 75 mg daily, and told me it would make me calmer immediately. He also said that within a week it would restore my filter mechanisms, which would make me feel less merged with other people. I was pleased. It had been a lot to go through to get the drug I needed, but at least I had finally got it. Paul went home and I realized that I had not eaten a single thing all day. I was presented with possibly the worst dinner I had ever had in my life – unidentifiable meat and pasta so overcooked that it had turned to glue, but I was so hungry that I ate it all. I telephone Jaina to say that I could not make her son's first birthday party that evening and she passed on the message to Janice, who came to visit me that evening. It was good to see her. For the first time in ages I did not feel threatened by her. In some way, in this awful place, for the first time in six months, I felt safe.

A week passed, sometimes quickly, sometimes agonizingly slowly. I had never felt so lonely, and yet there were times when everything seemed to be mending. Paul came up every day to visit and we went out for long walks. The June weather was beautiful and I often sat outside with Sybil and Stella, the two young patients who had become, and remain to this day, my friends. The nurses did not talk to us but we talked endlessly to each other, letting our imaginations run riot and learning how to have fun again. One day the three of us went out for an invisible picnic, a wonderful antidote to the hospital food. At night we would stand at the windows watching the lights of Blackheath, which we called 'the magic city'. I could say anything to them, no matter how bizarre. We were comfortable with each other in a way I had not been with other people for so long.

There was little to do on the ward. There was a doctor's meeting once a week where the psychiatrist presided over the group of patients. No one talked.

'Well, if no one's going to say anything,' said the psychiatrist, 'you must all be okay, so we'll finish the meeting.'

Aside from this there was an occupational therapy assistant who asked me if I would like to go to Tesco's with her and join in a cooking group. She did not know I was an OT. Oddly, my cooking skills were one of the few things that had not deteriorated. I declined her offer.

The ward round did not take place until the following week. I walked into a room where fifteen people sat in a circle. I recognized only my psychiatrist, a junior doctor, a nurse from the ward and the OT assistant. The rest were strangers.

'Sit down', said my psychiatrist. 'Can you tell us – do you hear voices?'
'Can you tell me who all these people are?', I replied.
'*She shouldn't tell them too much*', said the voice. '*She should be selective.*'

The psychiatrist told me who everyone was. I told them very little. My chlorpromazine was increased to 300 mg daily and I was told I could go home on overnight leave.

I was in hospital for three weeks. Overnight leave went well. When I returned from weekend leave a nurse handed me a medication card.

'Go and get your prescription from pharmacy', she told me. 'You're discharged now.'
The psychiatrist told me to go back to work.
'You've had a major breakdown', she said. 'But you're not schizo-phrenic.'

But she recommended that I join the National Schizophrenia Fellowship anyway.

I went home. It was not bad. It was just that I felt like I was landing on earth from another planet. I felt like the astronauts who had returned from the moon and, having seen their world from afar, gone completely bonkers. I knew that I could not go back to work immediately so I got a sick note from my GP for four weeks. But the pressure started straight away. The staff at The Grange began to phone me.

'We really miss you, Jan.'
'We do hope you're going to come back soon.'
'We need to do a programme review and we really can't do it without you.'
Help, I thought.

I knew that The Arbours Association were renowned for dealing with psychotic patients and so I went for an assessment. I was cagey. I badly wanted help but felt that I was still too psychotic to be taken on, and my previous therapy had left me unconfident. Never mind my lack of confidence at being a manager of a day centre – I was not even confident of my ability to be a patient! Amazingly, so I thought, I was given an appointment to see a therapist with whom I could decide whether treatment was appropriate. In that first session she did not say much, but I cried and cried, and decided that, on some level, I must feel safe with her. I was very glad when she said she would see me three times a week. I knew that I had to try to understand what had happened to me, if I was to rebuild my life, cope with my role at work and prevent it happening again. Such understanding, though, was not to be quickly or easily come by.

Part 3: Professional patient/patient professional?

On 26 July I went back to work at The Grange. I deliberately chose a day when most of the clients and staff were on an outing so only two members of staff were around. They were very nice to me, welcomed me back and gave me a plant, but the gentle return was short lived. At the first staff meeting my team demanded a programme review, something which I knew always caused major conflict. I asked them to wait a month, until I was feeling stronger, but was bombarded from all sides.

'The review is due now – it has to happen *now*.'
'We've been two whole months without management.'
'We need *you* to organise this.'
'You have to get on with being a manager.'

In retrospect they were, of course, angry with me for abandoning them, but at this time I was not in a position to analyse their behaviour. All I could feel was guilt, inadequacy, and a sense that I had done something wrong which I had to put right.

There was a new client group, younger people with very different needs, and also there was a lot of competitive strife between the day centre and residential teams. Everyone had different needs and I did not feel I could meet any of them. All I felt confident in was sitting with clients in informal one-to-ones, but no one was going to let me get away with that! The prevailing attitude was 'business as usual' and there was no one I could talk to, no one with whom I felt I could admit that I just was not coping. The more I felt overwhelmed the more pressure I got.

'Jan – you have to take more of a lead in the meetings.'

'Jan – we're being under-managed.'

For the first time in my life I dreaded going to work. I was tearful and nauseous much of the time. Often I vomited in the morning when it was time to go to work. Also, for the first time in my career I remember feeling a profound distinction between clients and staff. 'Us' and 'Them'. I realized that I now felt more comfortable with the clients than with the staff.

No one realized how serious my breakdown had been, but of course this was because I had never told them. Now it was impossible. If I tentatively began to say how bad I was feeling the pressure just increased. The message I always received was: 'Jan, you have to be well. You have to look after us.'

By mid-November the situation was becoming intolerable and I had a week off sick. The voice was back:

'She hasn't got the guts to kill herself. She's no good. It'd be easier for everyone if she was dead.'

I began to feel unsafe with Paul again, not wanting to go out, isolating myself. I decided I needed to apply for redeployment, to a less demanding job, but obviously this could not happen straight away. In the meantime I requested some outside support, which was refused by higher management.

One evening, as I was in the bath, the voice persisted and persisted.

'She should drown herself. She should drown herself.'

I put my head under the water and tried to keep it there. Of course I came up spluttering but I realized that things were getting out of hand, to say the least. It was time to go back to my GP, who confirmed my fears.

'You need to go back to hospital', she told me.

Back in hospital things were very different. There was no Sybil and Stella, for a start. There were, however, lots of angry young men. The nurses spent their time shut in the office and the door to the ward was locked most of the time. There was much overt racism among the staff. Later I found out that one of the nurses had been badly assaulted by one of the patients, and so the staff were very scared. I was scared; the nurses were scared – it could hardly be a therapeutic environment. This time there was a qualified OT on the ward but she avoided me and whenever I spoke to her she seemed very nervous and unsure. Was she scared of me as well?

What the stay did give me, however, was 400 mg of chlorpromazine, which made it much, much easier to engage in psychotherapy. For the first time I felt able to talk about hearing the voice. Finally I managed also to tell the psychiatrists.

'Sometimes I do hear a voice', I said. 'But I didn't feel able to tell you before.'
'Oh of course we knew all along', smiled the doctor.
So it was true. People could read my thoughts!

I decided it was better not to return to The Grange and had, in all, six months off work, during which time I organized my redeployment – a community OT post with physically disabled people. During this time I wrote to the manager at Goodmayes and asked to see my hospital notes.

'Diagnosis unclear', it read. 'Strong personality element.'

That was worrying. I knew about personality disorders and how difficult they are to treat. But then again, I did not feel like I was a personality disorder.

Though I was very nervous about going back to work, after the first week I soon found my feet and began to feel a new confidence in my abilities. Because I was new, and not a manager, there was no pressure either to know everything or to take control. I also received lots of positive feedback, which seemed surprising. I had got so used to people telling me I couldn't do my job properly.

Over the next 18 months my confidence grew and slowly I became more motivated and energetic. Paul and I had a good holiday in Morocco and I managed to reduce the chlorpromazine from 400 mg to 200 mg daily with no ill effects. Yes, sometimes the voice still had to have its say, but now this centred around my psychotherapy, where it seemed my madness was being contained. I knew now that the voice was a part of me, but if I could keep it safely compartmentalized in my psychotherapy sessions then I could get on with the rest of my life.

During this period someone asked me to join a working party for day care, organized by Newham MIND, and so began my involvement with MIND, which has continued and become a valuable part of my support network. Working for MIND also made me increasingly aware that I was missing mental health work, and I felt just about ready to return. I was also, surprisingly, finding myself increasingly frustrated by not being a manager. When I saw an advertisement for Head OT at Redbridge Health Care Trust I was initially reticent. I imagined it would be based at

Goodmayes and therefore not quite the standard I was looking for! But it was not based at Goodmayes and it was about mental health care and was a management post. I applied for the job. I was somehow convinced that if I worked for Redbridge I would never have to go back to Goodmayes again. Also, unconsciously, I had a need to put things right. Part of me wanted to make the hospital better.

I got the job but naturally they required a report from my psychiatrist. I went to see her.

> 'If I became unwell again, I wouldn't have to go back to Goodmayes, would I?' I asked hopefully.
> 'Mmm', she said. 'Could be a problem – East Ham Memorial never has any beds, Claybury's out of the question as you'll be working with patients from there, and St Clements is horrid.'
> 'So?', I said.
> 'Don't you like Goodmayes?', she asked me.
> I skirted.
> She laughed.
> 'Well, just don't get ill again', she said.
> I said I would try not to.

I was surprised to get the job. Although I knew I could do it I felt sure I would fail the medical, but in November 1993 I began. Initially it was very strange. Although I was not based at Goodmayes I still had to go there for meetings and it was very odd walking through the door as a professional. In one of the meetings I met the OT who had been on the ward when I was a patient, the one who had looked so scared of me. She was still very uneasy in my presence and avoided talking to me. This was a problem that obviously needed sorting out professionally. So we went to someone's leaving party, got extremely drunk, and had a good old chat. It was amazing to find out that she had been terrified of me on the ward as she thought I would be judging her OT practice. I assured her that it really had been the *last* thing on my mind.

Over the next two years things went smoothly. Of course I had off days, like everyone does. My off days, I suppose, differed from other people's in that I heard a voice in my head. But this voice was now benign, merely echoing my thoughts. It did not stop me from enjoying my life for I suppose I had become accustomed to it. I was enjoying my job, working voluntarily for MIND, having a good social life and Paul and I had a wonderful holiday in India. I became more aware of what pressures triggered the voice, of what I should avoid. I became more able to say no.

But of course you cannot always avoid pressure, nor mete it out in tolerable doses. Christmas 1995 was a bad time. Paul's mother was dying; my line manager at work was about to leave and the committee at Newham MIND were engaged in conflict which I was being asked to sort out. Moreover there were problems within my own family, between my parents and my sister, which I was becoming increasingly drawn into. I began to feel uneasy again.

Now a second voice had developed, a voice I did not recognize: the other side of the telephone conversation. In some ways it was easier to hear the full conversation, but the content was hardly reassuring.

> '*She's selfish.*'
> '*Yes, she is.*'
> '*She doesn't care about her family.*'
> '*No, she should be doing more, shouldn't she?*'
> '*Yes, she should.*'

I was slipping back into the other world. Again things took on strange significance; rules came into play which frightened me. In psychotherapy I became very aware of how my therapist sat; what she did with her hands affected me. For example if she sat with her arms folded everything was fine. If she touched her face or clasped her hands it meant I would be destroyed. Outside I worried about scarves. Anyone wearing a scarf meant danger for me. It was winter. There were lots of scarves about. The world was a very dangerous place. And I could hear people talking about me on the bus, commenting on my appearance, on what I was wearing. Also at this time I began to smell a pervasive stench of decay, of rotting flesh. The smell followed me everywhere, constantly. I knew that it was not real, that it was only *like* a smell, but I could smell it all the same and it was disgusting. The voices were getting louder and I was having to cover up, being careful at work not to look round and respond to them.

Then, one night in the bath, I had the radio plugged into the mains and turned up loud. I could still hear the voices over the music.

> '*It would be better if she was dead.*'
> '*Nothing's worked so far.*'
> '*If we erase her thoughts and put our own in it would work.*'
> '*Yes, we can make her put the radio in the bath.*'
> '*That would work.*'
> '*Yes, we'll make her do that.*'

I remember crying out, 'No!' I was terrified. I knew then for sure that I was very unwell.

Fortunately I had a scheduled outpatient appointment and my psychiatrist asked if I would like to go back into hospital. I knew I was not safe and at this stage I did not even care that it was back to Goodmayes. This time, however, it was much better. For a start I had my own room, and I was assured that this was not because I worked for the Trust! The nursing staff were much kinder, explaining everything that was going on, and there was none of the overt racism like before. The OT on the ward was in a support group I ran at work but I had thought to ask my boss to warn her that I was coming in. She was fine with me. The other staff I worked with were not around on the ward but they did come to visit me in the evenings and were very supportive and caring. There was no pressure to go back to work, just to get myself well. It was from one of my visitors that I learned a surprising thing – that one of the keys on my large bunch was actually the key to the ward! It felt good, although I am not sure that my psychiatrist would have approved. I did not really think that the nurses were going to lock me in against my will, but it was reassuring to know that I could get out if they did. I think it illustrates well a paradox of mental health care: the need for containment without imprisonment – a fine line.

For the first time I was given droperidol, the 'don't give a fuck' drug, which calmed me considerably. It was not that it made any of the symptoms go away – it was just that I did not care about them any more. That, together with 650 mg chlorpromazine, ensured that I was well and truly doped up. But I felt okay. I was safe.

My discharge was well planned and I felt, all in all, I had received a better service. In my last ward round I was asked, according to the care programme approach, what I wanted. What I really wanted was for them to pay my psychotherapy fees, but I did not ask. I was offered family therapy, an option that, after careful consideration and advice from friends, I chose not to take up. But it may be an option in the future.

Home again I felt disorientated but my recovery was quicker than before and I knew I would get the support I needed when I returned to work. It was not easy. Both my concentration and motivation were affected, but my manager and staff team were prepared to make every allowance. Everyone was adamant that I must not overdo it, I must go home if I ever felt bad, and I must talk when I needed to. Moreover the clear message was that I did not have to be perfect. Without that pressure I was able to regain my confidence.

So now I am a mental health professional again. Who knows if I shall change my hat yet again and become a mental health patient? Statistics would say that hospital readmission is likely for schizophrenics, but then I have always been told that I am not schizophrenic. No one really knows what to call me. All I am clear about is that I have a tendency to slip into another world, the other world where the rules are very different and very frightening. My psychotherapy is now about discovering the meaning of this strange world and the meaning of its rules.

I have a tremendous support network: Paul, my friends, my family, my women's group at Newham MIND. I try to balance an active social life with enough time on my own. Painting and drawing have been integral in allowing me to express the terrors that cannot be verbalized.

It is certainly the case that my experience has made me a better practitioner. I think that I was a good practitioner before I went mad, but I know now that I am less coercive, that I give people more choice. I am more aware of doing things *with* people, not *to* them, because my experience has made me realize that people who are in a different reality still have enormous capabilities.

Nowadays I make a more conscious effort to maintain good boundaries. Having been without boundaries myself, I know how important they are. Perhaps for me, because the distinction between professional and patient is not so strong, I need to make a bigger effort. It is important for me, when I am in my professional role, to provide consistency and strength for those I am supporting. I don't want them to worry about me, but, again, I don't want to create unnecessary barriers. Perhaps the notion of having established boundaries, not barriers, conveys a sense of what I mean. Also, my boundaries between work and home are stronger.

It is not now so uncommon for ex-users of psychiatric services to work in the field. I know a lot of ex-users who claim to know what is best for people, having experienced madness themselves. My feeling is that my experience has certainly given me insight into the concept of other worlds, but that is not for one moment to say that I can understand anyone else's other world. I would not presume that any two psychoses are the same. What is so frightening about psychosis is the fact that no one else can ever understand it fully. I have certainly been on both sides of the fence, but I will never know the ultimate truth.

In some ways I am stronger. In others not. My sense of self, I think, is now not so strong because I know it can be eroded in such a big way. Paradoxically I have a stronger sense of my own fragility. I think little about the future. The present is hard enough. This is for me, perhaps, not so hard because of being epileptic for so many years. You learn that you might set off for the shops but you can never be sure of getting there. What I have learned most of all is to enjoy the present.

Epilogue

At work I am doing a painting group with two very psychotic patients, Mary and Bella. They do not know that I have been in hospital. I would tell them if they asked me directly but they do not. The reason I do not tell my clients is that I am paid to give them support and I want them to feel that support is safe and solid. If I thought it would help anyone to tell them, I would not hesitate.

Mary is painting an elephant.
'This elephant fucked me', she says. 'I had its baby.'
Bella is murmuring quietly to the voices which only she can hear.
'Jan', Mary says suddenly. 'You've had a hard time in your life, haven't you?'
I do not need to say anything.
'Yes', says Bella, joining in. 'Jan's been out of this world.'
They both smile at me. It feels good.

Chapter 4
Fire and Ice

CATHY CONROY

Editorial

Mania affords the viewer a special perspective of the human universe – both internally and consensually. Although we once accepted the dramatic basis of the madness narrative, psychology has progressively stripped the soul out of the psyche, in its pursuit of a scientific model of human functioning. Indeed, for the centuries that psychiatry has now told the story of human experience, it has increasingly robbed those stories even of their innate drama and poetry in the retelling, or translation. But the dimensions of human experience are, by definition, dramatic, and Cathy Conroy's story emphasizes the drama of her own lifeworld, redressing the balance, to some extent, reminding us of the poetics of the experience of madness. Indeed, she takes us even further, helping us to appreciate how the human narrative may be underpinned by a musical score.

Cathy Conroy's chapter offers a special challenge to the received view of madness. There is little holding back in her writing, as there appears to be in her life. Cathy celebrates her mania and depression as an integral part of her creative drive towards a new selfhood. Or, it might be more appropriate to say that Cathy celebrates the function of her experience, serving for her as one of the core props for her creative process.

Cathy Conroy is, however, no idle romantic. She knows, intimately, the distress associated with mania and depression; she has sought, and continues to seek, ways of living with and through such experiences. At the same time she is clearly ambivalent about losing the connection with the infinite, which mania and depression have afforded her. She seems to suggest that there is always a price to pay for any wisdom and, so far, she is willing to continue to pay the price of her journey towards her own enlightenment.

This story offers complex challenges to the professional reader. In some respects Cathy Conroy is an ordinary woman: wife, mother and part-provider

54

to her home and family. She is also a poet and musician. Traditionally, we try to split off such 'creative types', as if they are, in some way, different from the rest of us who fall into the Slough of Despond, or worse. Yet, a careful reading of Cathy's story suggests that her voice may well be the voice of the majority, if not of Everyman. In 'Fire and Ice' she may be illustrating how much of the experience of psychic distress is common, but often needs an uncommon voice to express it. More importantly, Cathy's story might worry us about our assumption that the point of mental health services is to eradicate the experience of distress. The prospect of silencing the voice of 'Fire and Ice' could never be taken lightly; the songbirds are already vanishing from our sight and hearing. 'Fire and Ice' is, in many respects, a sorrowful song, but sorrow has its healing properties, as well as its pain. The leap to 'cure' might also carry the penalty of forgetting, something that Cathy appears reluctant to do.

★   ★   ★   ★   ★

How can words depict perfumed valleys, dancing daphne and lavender, feathered ferns, sun-drenched dreams, leaping heart, harmonies of rapture?

How can words even begin to convey the experience of what it is like to live with a bipolar disorder? What words will speak to matters of the heart, intense at times, so marvellously sweet and so desperately sad?

My life has been shaped by tremendous mood swings. I have found myself revelling in the glory and delight of nature, being transported and transfixed; seeing dark clouds impede my vision as I have wrestled with intense sadness and feelings of volatile anger and irrational madness, disabling me and casting black shadows amidst me and my loved ones.

I will never forget the first intense mood swings I experienced. I was seventeen and was walking to my boarding school in the country, after an English lesson. My sense of union with nature overwhelmed and transported me. The splendid nature of the universe, and particularly an apple tree, took on a significance that was mystifying. That night sleep would not come. Rising, I stared out of a window at the black night and stayed there until dawn. I was overcome by these two simple experiences. They were also two forms of experience that would, in time, deepen in complexity and consequence. This had been my first intimation of epiphany.

If only these enduring and intense, but essentially gentle experiences had been the limit of my swings. As the years passed, the simple warning signs – heightened awareness, over-talkativeness, lack of sleep, intense emotion, over-spending, expansive thoughts – stampeded, untamed, into the full-blown chaos of manic experiences. My first psychotic breakdown occurred in 1978, while I was teaching a class of third graders. Events in the classroom became hectic as I asked for hundreds of things to be achieved by the children. We were flying kites while singing 'let's go fly a kite', we were painting, reciting poetry, making massive projects and creating plays at break-neck speed.

In the nights my husband clung on to me perplexed, wondering what the hell was happening. I lay sleepless. Terrible nightmares with religious connotations filled my head in the hours of sleep I did have. Then there were grandiose thoughts and excited, revelatory feelings. I went from a general hospital to a psychiatric hospital to another psychiatric hospital. I left the last with 36 tablets to take per day. I had no insight into the course of events. How could I, since no discussion had provided me with the slightest understanding of this nightmare whirlwind.

At home, days merged into each other meaninglessly and relentlessly. I was like a zombie for months, in depression and a stupefying daze. An old friend came to stay with me – she'd just spent a year travelling overseas. She played scrabble with me day in, day out. I think I just made two- and three-letter words. It was the best I could do for months. My sister at Medical School tried to explain the nature of manic depressive psychosis, and so began the long move away from thinking that prescribed tablets were the sole cause of my strange illness and the months and months off work.

The appalling dark melancholia, the aching and crying were like an eternity. I longed for sleep. The emptiness and ghastliness described by Job haunted me:

> For the thing which
> I greatly feared is come upon me
> and that which I was afraid of
> Is come unto me
> I was not in safety, neither
> had I rest, neither was I quiet
> yet trouble came.
>
> (Job 3: 25–26)

And yet, all of this was such a contrast with another side of myself, the side of 'High Flight' described in John Magee's poem:

Oh! I have slipped the surly bonds of Earth
And danced the skies on laughter-silvered wings;
Sunward I've climbed and joined the tumbling mirth
of Sun-split clouds – and done a hundred things
You have not dreamed of – wheeled and soared and swung
High in the Sunlit silence.

(Magee, 1942)

Eighteen months after my first breakdown, the birth of my daughter, Jacinta, took place, followed by the birth of my first son, Bernard.

Miraculously, there was some time of stability and remission. I was able to do an Associate Diploma in Creative Arts in Music and spend long hours in the sun with my dear husband and children and with friends, relatively carefree, sleeping through most nights, rejoicing and celebrating.

Joseph, our third child, was born to Mozart's Sinfonia Concertante K364, in 1987. The pregnancy was fearful and throughout it I was teaching at a Technical and Further Education College, also teaching music at a preschool. However, the gift of sleep was now taken from me. In the depths of night after night I dragged myself from room to room, desperately trying to find rest and comfort without waking the family. I remember turning to the music of the St Louis Jesuits and the words in one of their hymns resonated with my mental state. I held fast to it:

> you shall cross the barren desert but you shall not die of thirst. You shall wander far in safety though you do not know the way.... You shall speak your words to foreign men and they will understand. You will see the face of God and live. (Isaiah 43:2–3)

I lived, but only just ! Two days after Joseph's birth I had a post partum psychosis. I was emotionally stripped, with nearly every feeling that is part of the human condition wrung out of me. The angel of death came to me and I was beset with a sickening fear. These were days of defeat, despair and a deep, dark wrenching of my self.

In a most unwell state, psychotic and dishevelled, I tucked Joseph into my shirt and fled through the park to our home, nearby. There was an uproar. I found dozens of ribbons and tied them into my daughter Jacinta's long, curly hair. In my mind she was a princess. For Bernard, my son, a national holiday was declared and little Joseph lay disconnected from me. At no point had the fragile bonds begun to wrap us together.

My sister came to stay. I bathed often with my guardian angel beside me. In deep worry, my husband made veiled telephone calls and the crisis team made plans. In Calvary Hospital, in Canberra, I was without my family and without my new baby. The psychiatric ward was directly below the obstetrics ward. I stared at all the babies through the glass. On an intellectual level, thoughts were spiralling. Emotionally I was as dead as a doorknob. A beloved friend breast-fed Joseph for me and then my sister-in-law took over the task. After several weeks Joseph was brought to the hospital so we could be together. I was heartbroken that I could not breast-feed Joseph. The lithium prevented that. I distinctly recall my inability patiently to give Joseph a bottle and go through all the baby procedures. I sensed and understood the nurses' frustration, but I also wondered how they could denigrate me. My God, here was I in a stricken situation that was beyond my control. Nonetheless, I was given a great deal of freedom with Joseph in that hospital and each day I bundled him into the pram and pushed him around for hours, disconnectedly with a gulf as big as Carpentaria between us.

Initially when I came home, days were just as nightmarish, as I slipped in and out of reality. It was taking so long to feed Joseph with a bottle. I recall, one day, expecting him to feed from a teaspoon. My family assessed the situation. I was in a deep unknown. For so long now I had awaited the pinking dawn, its rosy luscious beauty. Alas, no elated feelings of anticipation, just a mind of dead tree-trunk – aridity. There were glimmers of aching and disenchantment, but mostly my inside was like a corpse.

Months rolled by in a blur. I remember being disappointed by advice not to return to teaching at the Child Care Studies Unit until I was really well. Another setback. So much was my identity related to my ability to work; or to how others perceived me.

We took a trip to New Zealand and I watched Jacinta and Bernard and my husband Gerry lovingly talk to, play with and cuddle Joseph. I saw his responsive gaze, his magnificent placid but alert disposition and in the depths of my soul some life stirred. At the same time I was praying to the Lord. One night I felt a strange, joyous intoxication as my cry to the heart of the universe felt heard:

Searching beyond horizons
& past long cast shadows
Dreaming ocean salt spray, depths unfathomed
Beholding string clouds, whisking spun moondust
Still unquenched thirst of you darling charged mystery
Rocked, swathed rolling in awesome might, maker. (C. Conroy)

Depression slowly diminished and hope gradually returned. I began to complete my Bachelor of Education degree and embarked on a new full-time job, as a social educator with intellectually disabled adults. Entering the realm of people whose perceptual and conceptual abilities are so different from ours required a new way of thinking, of seeing and of being. It was at this time that my sister Bernadette and I had the glorious opportunity of meeting Jean Vanier. He was on a lecture tour from Trosly-Breuil in France. His life has been spent in building community with the intellectually disabled. With powerful words and a tender heart he called forth in me a special way of appreciating the intellectually disabled.

In 1987, in the wake of the Richmond Report (State Health, 1983), intellectually disabled people at Kenmore Hospital Goulburn (Southern New South Wales) were separated from mentally ill people. They still shared the same beautiful grounds with magnificent oriental plane trees, chestnuts, pines, elms, beeches and eucalypts; beds of jonquils, daphne, camellias and agapanthus. One day the other social educator and I took a small group of these people on an outing. It was such a memorable day, such a luminous, polished and utterly perfect day. In my mind it is still 'East Grove Driving' day and the recollection of it has remained joyous.

> I take centuries for myself
> to catch and hold the elusive rays
> blazing brilliance.
>
> I'm traversing new land now and
> the human time is all the time
> but the eternal marks no time.....
>   it holds
>   it holds
> Astonishing glory still/stopped
> gold shafted light curling and reforming
> in floating wisdom
> Gasp in awe
> breathtaking spread of enlightened land
> colours colluding, catching up heaped offering of heaped heart
> Leaves fashioned and unfathomed –
> shiver, tremble; a new universal song seeds. (C. Conroy)
>
> He maketh peace in thy borders,
> and covers thee with the finest of the wheat. (Psalm 147:14)

While working with intellectually disabled people, I would sometimes meet people with mental illness and I would feel particularly drawn to them, perhaps because of my own mental illness. When the opportunity to work as an advocate for the mentally ill arose in August 1994, the encouragement of my family and friends, and a deep 'in-the-bones' interest, inspired me. I had in the back of my mind Shakespeare's words in the *Tragedy of Julius Caesar:*

> There is a tide in the affairs of men,
> Which taken at the flood, leads on to fortune;
> Omitted, all the voyage of their life
> Is bound in shallows and in miseries
> On such a full sea are we now afloat,
> And we must take the current when it serves,
> Or lose our ventures.

Having had the opportunity of employment in a number of stimulating and interesting positions, I believe I have an acute sense of the alienation suffered by many as a result of their mental illness or disability. As a teacher, I worked with a wide variety of students stigmatized as a result of their experience and, as a social educator of intellectually disabled adults, stories of wounded minds and hearts were constantly evident.

The journey of the mentally ill is often inward, burrowing into states of being where personal worthlessness, isolation, desolation and a sense of unconnectedness prevail. Although opportunity to achieve in the world of work may exist, there still remains stigma designed by others but cradled within.

Living knowledge of such stigma resulted in a burning desire to advocate on behalf of those with mental illness. The fire behind such a calling is rekindled for me each time I see how my present, valued social role is not shared by a large number of people with mental illness in hospital. People who are not seen as having valued social roles are considered to be of essentially low value. People seen in such a light have very different life experiences from those in valued roles, and are likely to be rejected, persecuted, and treated in ways which tend further to diminish their dignity, adjustment, growth, competence, health, wealth, lifespan, etc. Such treatment will largely express and reflect the devalued societal roles they are 'playing'.

How a person is perceived and treated by others will determine strongly how that person subsequently behaves. Therefore, the more consistently a person is perceived and treated as being in a negative role, the more likely it is that she/he will conform to that expectation and actually will behave in ways that are not valued by society. On the other hand, the more a person is encouraged to assume roles and behaviours which are appropriate and desirable, the more will be expected of him/her, and the more she/he will live up to those positive roles.

I think that a turning point for me was in realizing this, seeing the greatest human potential as the ability of each one of us to empower and acknowledge the other, to empathize. Just by being there, by talking to people, by being comfortable with my own label, I can contribute to positive health promotion, understanding and advocacy. To have myself 'felt the wind of the wing of madness' has been enlightening in these circumstances.

In the psychiatric hospital I have met many immensely brave people. Sometimes they have seemed overwhelmed by guilt, internal conflict and insecurity. As an advocate my role is to protect the rights and the welfare, sometimes even the lives of these people.

It is good to acknowledge the other when they face confusion, loss, disorientation and disheartenment.

> The process of healing and growth is immensely quickened when the sun of another's belief is freely given ... time and place in the sunshine [is an apt] metaphor [for] the ... stimulus for ... psychological ... transformation. (Houston, source unknown)

As a person moves away from the acute episode of their mental illness, I sometimes introduce a time of story-telling, which might go like this:

> One day at my beloved 'Braeside', I wandered off. I went through a number of the back paddocks, alongside the cottage paddock, past the windmill and beyond the caves. Then I realized how late and how dark it was. I was lost. I was alone. There were thousands of tussocks to trip over. It was a time of fear. Deep fear. I was put in hospital because I had become separated from myself and from others. I had become lost in the long yellow tussocks of my past and my present. I was alone in the tussocks. (Frame, 1980)

I find such metaphors useful, at least as useful as the metaphor of 'mental illness', which suggests that the locus of one's difficulties is, like other illnesses, in an individual's body. There are accounts of a person's 'breakdown' beyond the psychiatric. It is misleading to locate a person's lived experience just in their one, individual body (Barker, 1995). As a consumer advocate I can use narratives like the one above to help convey to people a more inclusive picture and a more authentic story of what has happened to them and their part in it. I believe that, to do this effectively, I have to have an ecological vision of individual human and social development, social education and society.

I want to see such a vision reflected in statutory mental health services – individual reflection about who and what people are in their lives, organizational reflection as to the purpose of that organization in the community. Such reflection should explore the interplay between self, service and community.

Carlos Castaneda (1968), in *The Teachings of Don Juan* says:

> Any path is only a path, and there is no affront, to oneself or to others, in dropping it if that is what your heart tells you.... Look at every path closely and deliberately. Try it as many times as you think necessary. Then ask yourself, and yourself alone, one question.... Does this path have a heart? If it does, the path is good; if it doesn't it is of no use.

When there is an opportunity for modelling new possibilities, for different *illuminated* paths, paths with heart, true exploration of our predicament can take place. In Nelson Mandela's inaugural speech, he claimed: 'Our deepest fear is not that we are inadequate. Our deepest fear is that we are powerful beyond measure. It is our light, not our darkness, that most frightens us.' Such insight springs from anguish, wounding, stigma, alienation in single rooms, labels, suffering, altered consciousness, desolation and betrayals. But it is an insight eventually leading to triumph. Advocacy can help a person in his/her expression of this powerful light.

An active and vigorous advocacy service is a logical and just outcome of the last decade's movement of the mentally ill away from institution-based care and back to lives that are as fulfilling and productive as possible, in a community setting and in the context of community-based care. The full acceptance of advocacy as a 'normal' activity within the mental health services will, it is hoped be the natural (and properly resourced) upshot of deinstitutionalization and other changes in the culture of statutory mental health care.

Ideological rhetoric about 'participation', 'consumer consultation' and 'collaborative care' means very little, though, if the ability to represent oneself is hobbled. The advocate's role in empowering individuals to become successful self-advocates often involves supporting them in their early attempts to be heard and, if necessary, speaking for them. A major part of the advocate's brief is to enable the client to attain the skills, autonomy and confidence to be able to defend his/her rights and dignity him/herself, without the need of an advocate. Without this focus, advocacy can become yet another disempowering hurdle placed in the path of those already labouring under many disadvantages.

The idea that mental health consumers can and should be responsible partners in their own treatment and rehabilitation plans is still a radical view, but is becoming mainstream in some countries. The education and utilization of clients as advisers within mental health services, and payment for their participation in these capacities, is an essential part of a participatory and consultative service.

Recently a person suffering from Munchausen's Syndrome came to Kenmore hospital. His is a 20 year history of self-harm and mutilation. He was maligned, intensely disliked and marginalized. He moved between the Base Hospital, where he needed medical attention, and the psychiatric hospital. He hated Kenmore and Kenmore said that it had nothing to offer him. On the day of his departure, he attended a Tribunal. We had discussed at length his desire to leave the hospital. I was concerned for his welfare if he left now: many things were unresolved and even if there were no effective 'treatment' on offer, for him just to be in a place of safety seemed important. Paul agreed for me to plead with the Tribunal to have him stay longer, for it was my belief that 'the moral treatment of those we routinely label "untreatable" requires more than the application of static ethical principles. The traditional virtues of compassion, humility, and fidelity are an often-neglected dimension of ethical responsibility... '(Christensen, 1995).

I saw, in my role as advocate, that there *were* some things that could be done for Paul. I made a tape of the most sensuous and lovely music I could think of, including some of the tracks I knew Paul loved.

One day, while listening to music together, I asked him to close his eyes and to visualize his heart, and then to see his son's heart contained inside his heart. I asked him to put his hands on his heart and to imagine his heart and his son's heart surrounded by a world heart. Just before the music began, I asked him: 'Have you told yourself lately that you love you....? And then we listened... (Van Morrison and the Chieftains 'Have I told you lately that I love you?')

The Tribunal listened to the psychiatrists, doctors, nursing unit manager, case manager and legal-aid solicitor and to Paul. My pleas, though, were disregarded. The decision was made in response to a doctor who callously documented twenty years of Paul's tormented life. Jeffery Masson says that it is only the truly 'healthy' who see through the pretence of psychiatry in the institution. I was certainly feeling dangerously healthy.

That night Paul was sped to Sydney to the Matthew Talbot Hostel, a free person, a person proclaimed to be not mentally ill. In deep need and inner anguish again that evening, he ripped his stomach open with a knife.

'Compassion impels us to stand with our clients and take seriously the reality of their pain and confusion' (Christensen, 1995), not disregard them, fob them off, boot them out because they are too expensive and submerged at the bottom of an overfull basket. We wash our hands of people too easily, Pontius Pilate style, when, after all, we are supposedly equal in the sight of God.

Let us picture ourselves huddled together, closely united – like a tree in the middle of a huge bush-fire that has swept through the timberland; a tree blackened and charred, with brown, scorched leaves and with bark singed and peeling; yet flowing through the centre is rich sap, and sunk deeply in the earth are roots barely touched, sheltering and revivifying. Like the tree enduring the flames, we the patients, and we the staff and the services catering for them, have the capacity for regeneration and renewal.

The tree might symbolize our own marvellous, creative urge to promote a more enlivened mental health system; connected branches, networking, outstretched and yielding, bearing great fruit and nourishing to hearts, minds and souls.

Seven months ago, elements of all my previous breakdowns tumbled back together into another one. I went to mass sixteen times in a row, three times on Sunday. My preoccupation and all-embracing passion was for union with the Anima Christi. While the rest of the family were away at a folk festival, Bernard came to mass with me on Easter Sunday. I was so malleable, I think he sensed I needed a 'bodyguard'. In these last years in breakdown Joseph has always partially accepted the role of my caretaker. Once when he was six and I was unwell and driven, he delighted in taking me to his hideout in the park. I ventured much further with him, collecting some intellectually disabled adult friends. I took them to 'Fibre Design', a lovely 'upmarket' Art and Craft place and, with great speed, charged very expensive skirts and hats and clothes to my credit card. We then proceeded as a group to the Paragon Café, for a party. The person from Fibre Design, noting my unusual manic state, called my husband. He came and joined in the party, saying the purchases were all wonderful, but 'not today darling'.

It is hard to imagine my life without its current depth of emotional intensity, forever having to tame my feelings and harness the depths of my longings, sublimating the urgency of my encounter, folding back – smoothing the rush and ache of my heart. Breakdown, the very first time, contains rich and strong spiritual memories. The remnants of these memories form a pattern, as if from an inner weaving, a carpeted mandala. The mandala's symbolism is of inner and outer connection. The richness of the textual design is not often discussed in mental health services. Most of the psychiatrists I have encountered while a mental health advocate have spent virtually no time on the *substance* of the mentally ill person's experience, its potential in working towards the development of inner emotional and spiritual connections. Patients' confused states are often treated with anti-psychotic medicines alone, and treated quite savagely.

Merleau-Ponty (1962) describes how we humanize our environment by coating it with dimensions of ourselves, 'and equally we make sense of our own indeterminate, transient feelings by embedding them in sensuous forms'. In many of my early hospitalizations, collage was an important part of my recovery. It seemed to offer me clarity, as I ripped pictures from magazines, assembling the fragments of photos and illustrations in a way that encapsulated my inner experience. The fragments formed symbols of my psychic world, emerging from the depths of inner caverns. The meanings I attributed have remained very important to me in understanding the patterns in my life contributing to my health and my illness.

So many means can be used for self-expression. Recently, while playing Corelli's La Folia, a Sonata featuring variations on an old Portuguese dance, some members of an acute ward began to trace their personal story lines. There was great interest in this activity. The desire to compose personal meaning was strong.

In *Real Presences* George Steiner (1992) says:

> ...it is in and through music that we are most immediately in the presence of the logical, the verbally inexpressible but wholly palpable energy in being, that communicates to our senses and to our reflection what little we can grasp of the naked wonder of life.

He adds, 'Music has celebrated the mystery of intuitions of transcendence'. Music too speaks to many, enabling them to untangle depths and perceive unspoken realms.

These words of rapture came to me in a recent state of union that progressed to psychosis:

Undress the golden tabernacle of my heart.
This tabernacle encrusted with miniature trees of the Universe
Dripping apple, holding kumquat, vermilion grape, lemon and pear,
Undress the golden tabernacle and behold the beholden... (C. Conroy)

At the time of this breakdown Joseph, now ten, embraced me with tenderness and special care. Our bond of love continues to tighten.

Some evenings I leave the acute ward, stepping out, overwhelmed by the immensity of the universe, most especially the stars in the darkened sky. I then contemplate the sometimes scarred lives within. Engulfed in reflection, there is at such times a sense of connection and rich exhilaration. It is possible to be lost in the depths, but one can also know there is something both within and outside, shrouding and protecting in its gentle darkness.

Oh time you snuck out and hid so artfully again
in misted moonbeams and long lost leafy elms
You crept out and we enshrouded in time beyond time
rejoiced in multitude jewelled joy and perplexed promises.
Newest myths of each, silked and special in the spiralling dream
Listened, grasped, cherished, soared. (C. Conroy)

Here is the golden thread, the mystical experience of consolation, peace, joy, hope, a place where loving arises, where one's mental turmoil is transformed into peace and renewal.

I think that, for me, recovery is not really about the cessation of intense mood swings. My fractal life patterns demand that I discover a path through long cold months of painful loss of feeling, awaiting the season of shooting buds on a swelling heart, to melt the snow and ice. I think my heartache is best summed up in words spoken by George Steiner (1993) in an interview: 'We are haunted by the sense of a breach with the promise in ourselves, with the best possibilities within ourselves. That hauntedness perhaps is our guilt.' This captures profoundly for me something of what living with a bipolar illness means, where my twisted states of emotion and thinking at times become unbearable for me and my family. Working and delving, struggling with the possibilities that provide new promise of hope, recollection, music and insight, lightens the guilt and anguish. Lithium, because of its desensitizing effect, is hard to take and slays me at times. But in the good times I've come to the point of embracing Ken Wilbur's words from *No Boundary*:

> A person who is beginning to sense the suffering of life is, at the same time, beginning to awaken to deeper realities, truer realities. For suffering smashes to pieces the complacency of our normal fictions about reality, and forces us to become alive in a special sense – to see carefully, to feel deeply, to touch ourselves and our worlds in ways we have heretofore avoided. It has been said and truly I think, that suffering is the first grace. In a special sense, suffering is almost a time of rejoicing, for it marks the birth of creative insight. (Wilbur, 1985)

Creative insight: grant us this gift dear Lord. Watch over the branches of the tree of life, the family, the music and all those with mental illness.

References & Bibliography

Barker P (1995) The logic of experience: developing appropriate care through effective collaboration. Presentation to the 21st Annual Nurses Conference, Canberra. September,1995.

Castaneda C (1968) The Teachings of Don Juan. USA: Penguin.

Christensen RC (1995) Editorial: Taking issue – the ethics of treating the untreatable. Psychiatric Service 46(12).

Frame J (1980) Quoted by Barker PJ. The Logic of Experience. Developing appropriate care through effective collaboration. 21st Annual Nurses Conference, Canberra ACT, September 1995.

Houston J (n.d.) The Search for the Beloved Jeremy Archer. Source unknown.

Isaiah 43:2–3.

Magee JG Jr (1942) 'High Flight' in Flying, May.

Merleau Ponty M (1962) Phenomenology of Perception,quoted in Ross M (Ed) (1978) The Development of Aesthetic Experience – Curriculum Issues in Arts Education, Vol. 3. Oxford: Pergamon Press, pp 52–53.

Shakespeare W (1982) Illustrated Stratford Shakespeare. London: Chancellor Press, Act 4, Scene 3, Lines 218 – 224.

State Health (1983) Richmond Report: Inquiry into health services for the psychiatrically ill and developmentally disabled. Haymarket, NSW: State Health Publications.

Steiner G (1992) Real Presences. London: Faber & Faber.

Steiner G (1993) Literary criticism as an act of love. ABC Radio '24 Hours' March, p 46.

Wilbur K (1985) No Boundary. Boston & London: Shambhala, p 85.

Chapter 5
The Flight of the Phoenix

ED MANOS

Editorial

'The Flight of the Phoenix' is the story of a man who, in being touched by madness, reveals the extraordinary potential of human ordinariness. Ed's story has all the ingredients of human drama: a tight-knit parental home, with strong religious and family values, blighted by the trauma of a mother's mental illness that, ultimately, is revealed as an enduring feature of the whole family tree. The way Ed Manos wrestles with his life in the early years will ring bells for many others who have faced similar devils. How Ed emerged to rebuild his life and to rescue something of value from the many traumas of his experience goes to the very core of the aim of this book: revealing what can be transformed from the Ashes of Experience. By its simple nature, Ed's story should inspire others to see beyond their distress, discovering a new communion with others, and perhaps new ways of capitalizing on the experience of distress.

Ed Manos has gone on, like so many other contributors to this book, to develop a career as a mental health advocate. In that work he has illustrated the value of getting close to people in mental distress, of being useful in a fundamental human sense. Ed is characteristic of those advocates who work away quietly at the grass roots, slowly building the foundations of a new Jerusalem of mental health care, using what he regards as his 'common sense' in an uncommonly creative and healing way. More than a decade ago he began running medication management groups with patients in hospital wards, helping them to learn about the value and dangers of the drugs they were taking, often blindly. As he fostered this educational alliance with his peers, the professional staff watched, in bewilderment, through the glazed partition of the central office. The radical critic might easily form the view that people like Ed Manos were set to replace many of the professional services, having become highly knowledgeable and effective professional consumers (prosumers). What appears to be happening, instead, is that people like Ed Manos are developing new ways of working collaboratively with professionals and academics, to foster new models of practice, and also to grow a new consciousness about mental health: one that is inclusive rather than exclusionary in character.

The way that Ed Manos talks appreciatively of those who have helped him shows the value he puts on the sense of true community. The professional reader, it is hoped, will feel that, through his story, Ed is reaching out to all professional colleagues, making contact, looking for new collaborators. The lay reader may feel a sense of affinity with a man who has found compassion for his own predicament and has built on that self-awareness to reach out to others. Ed's story has few frills and no fancies but is, nonetheless, a story of regeneration.

★   ★   ★   ★   ★

Just over four-and-a-half years ago I had my first major bipolar cycle for almost sixteen years. Looking back, it was the stress at work and cracks which had appeared in my relationships, at home in particular, that led to yet another spell in hospital. I had been on lithium for almost twenty-five years and it seemed to be time to upgrade this. Having managed myself over all this time with the support only of medication, it seemed time to start seeing a therapist to look in particular at my relationship problems. My kids were experiencing problems from living in this crazy world and its effects were certainly telling on me. For probably the last four years, I had been aware of being in mixed states: I had kept seeing my psychiatrist every three months, but only to tinker with my medication, because of the costs of asking for any more than that. Notably, I had not been sleeping and that should have been a key for me, if not also for my fellow consumers who knew the signs only too well.

I had my first experience of mental illness in 1968, when I was about seventeen, and it was wholly unexpected. I was a senior in high school, I had a brand new car which I had worked for ever since I was a kid and I was enjoying a good social life, despite being shy, especially when it came to dating. Gradually, I started to have increasing feelings of paranoia and had problems verbalizing this, especially to mom and dad. My mom had had psychiatric problems for as long as I could remember, originating in a post-partum depression after my brother's birth in 1947. She had seven or eight lengthy hospitalizations in state hospitals and in those days she was labelled schizophrenic, like everyone else, and got little more than heavy doses of thorazine and stelazine. That was the environment I grew up in with my mom – a very subdued woman, owing to medication, but also a very loving and caring mother.

We were a religious family, Catholics, and when we moved from New York City my dad ended up working for the Catholic Church for more than four years. I recall that I was in the church school grounds when I had my first experience of paranoia. When it eventually dawned on my dad, it must have caused him a lot of extra stress, given that for more than twenty-five years he had been trying to cope with my mom's experience of psychiatric illness, trying all the time to get her back to something like a normal state. What I did not know then was that this paranoia was the beginnings of manic depression and that I was following in my mom's footsteps, so to speak. Sadly, she was never properly diagnosed, even up until the time she died in 1978. It is clear from my family tree that this is very much a genetic disposition and now my seventeen-year-old son has joined the clan, having had his first episode of depression and recently spiralled up into a manic phase. Hopefully things will be very different for him, compared with mom and me and other members of our clan.

After my first bout of depression, it was a quick week and a half of paranoia and fear, and then I was back into the groove. I did OK until 1971 when I was a college sophomore and, after a debilitating physical illness, had a very similar experience of depression. I left college, finished my work at home, and was then helpfully transferred to Colorado. I had always been a keen athlete and sports kept my depression at a minimum. I was planning to major in criminal justice, hoping to become a socially conscious cop. Until then, I had only been afflicted by bouts of depression. Now I had my first real bout of mania, due to the stress of combining my college work with working for a private detective agency as an armed guard at a condominium. I guess working from 10.00 pm until 6.00 am, then heading on to college, trying to catch some sleep here, there and anywhere, was a risky business. I ended up needing to be hospitalized. I did try getting some help from a counsellor, but was put on some of the heavier major tranquillizers, which precipitated more paranoia, especially as this experience echoed my mom's. However, my stay in hospital eventually ended. I had to return home, as mom had come down with terminal cancer.

After she died, I returned to school for the senior year. One more semester under my belt. Colorado was quite a party scene in those days and, sadly, I did not have the social support I needed to corral me. I spiralled up a second time, despite having done well in school. So, I had to quit school again. Three-and-a-half years of college behind me but still I had little understanding of what was going on.

I then experienced the post-mania 'downing' which kept me in my home for a good six months. I hid in my room, coming out only at night, gaining a lot of weight and taking little care of my appearance or my hygiene. Eventually, my dad could take little more of this and he somehow managed to get me over to the local mental health clinic. Fortunately, I found a very non-traditional psychologist to whom I took an immediate liking. Although I was still being diagnosed as schizophrenic and did not get on to lithium for some time, I started to come out of my shell and was able to get back to work, eventually dating my old high school sweetheart. Soon, I moved to Trenton, the state capital, and got back into security work. All went well for about a year but I still had many difficulties, especially a lot of denial.

I did not have any real success at the business of living with my mania and depression until 1973 when, through my dad's influence, I got into a very good hospital in Patterson, New Jersey, mainly through his connections with the Catholic Church. It was there that I began to address some of my real-life problems, aided greatly by the psychiatric nurses who were very young, very pretty and very knowledgeable. They spotted my feelings of anger and helped me express it more appropriately, working in conjunction with the recreational and occupational therapists. Over a three-week period I was taught the practice of yoga by one of the nurses, and the recreational therapist helped me vent my anger more appropriately through swimming, basketball and working on the heavy bag. It was not all a picnic though, and I still had lots of negative experiences with the psychiatrist who, unfortunately, was very much into mind games. This brought my paranoia even more to the surface, as well as some delusional stuff. Overall, the experience on that ward was wonderful and taught me much about myself.

Then I had a period of normalcy, which left me stable for about two-and-a-half years. However, since I had both a credit card and a car, when I shot up into hypomania I would often just up sticks and hit the road. Once I got as far as Columbus, Ohio, a twelve-hour drive from New Jersey. By the end of that particular jaunt, I had reached the point where my metabolism was speeding just as much as the car in which I was travelling. I was taken through the emergency clinic and ended up in the University of Ohio Hospital where, after some liquid thorazine, I was assigned to a very young doctor who was both a psychologist and a psychiatrist. In less than ten minutes she diagnosed me as manic depressive, got on the phone to my dad and began the business proper of establishing me on a lithium regime. I emerged back into the light six days later and after seven years in a schizophrenic wilderness, between the ages of seventeen and twenty-four, I finally had a diagnosis and some beginnings of an understanding as to what had been going on in my life.

It has not exactly been plain sailing since then. There have been many ups and downs since, but I have managed to build a life for myself and my family. I had met my wife-to-be at that point and we married in 1976. One of the key things which helped me stay on the track was the fact that I did not have the resources that my co-consumers had, and I was forced to deal with all my denial factors head on. Although I could not afford the therapists and all their fancy prices, I knew that I needed to get my head around this experience and get some support. So I started to attend self-help groups. Depression groups, as such, were not available at that time. So I went to AA groups, men's groups, anything that was free and would have me. Although I had no real idea what I was getting into, this was to be the big departure in my life.

When I reflect on those early days and my feelings about those times and those experiences, I often ask, 'Where was Ed in all of this?'. Throughout those years, clearly there was more than one Ed on the go. First of all there was the kind, gentle Ed that I tried to be no matter how ill I ever became. Even when I was in full-blown mania on a hospital ward, I would still be trying to help people. Often I would be running around madly helping anyone who needed it or would take it, much to the amazement of the staff. On reflection, I realize that that was where I made the career switch proper, having discovered my aptitude for helping as well as the rewards which it brought me. At the same time, there was also the angry, explosive, scary Ed who could burst through without warning. Lastly, there was the abandoned Ed, who represented me at my most vulnerable. All but a couple of my high school friends had dropped me which, of course, is not an unusual experience.

Gradually, I seemed to establish some kind of balance and order to my world, with the help of lithium, marriage and work. These served as great buffers for the seasonal disturbance that I still suffer from. When the medication does not work, I turn on my holistic approaches to the full. I can find peace by walking on the ocean shoreline, which is five blocks away from my home, or by riding my bike, or by spending time with my son. I have also come to value other supports and, in particular, have returned to the church, joining the Knights of St Columbus, an organization dedicated to helping the needy in our state and country. Here I have found a new dimension to the word 'peace', in the form of making another kind of contribution to society. This clearly fills another need in me. I still hope to get back to school to get that elusive Bachelors Degree. I still dream of going on to do my Masters. That would definitely satisfy me. Maybe then I could teach properly. Currently I lecture about ten times a semester as an adjunct instructor at the University of Medicine and Dentistry in New Jersey, in the Psychosocial Rehabilitation Department. I lecture on all aspects of the consumer movement, but still dream about doing that properly from the base of my Masters education.

Like all consumers and, I guess, people in general, I learned how to hide my real distress and real feelings. I learned how to manipulate everybody around me; in particular, professional staff. I, too, was being manipulated, however, by a psychiatric system that was as lacking in compassion as it was in wisdom. I was repeatedly told that I could never marry, could never have a normal relationship, could never father a normal child. I was told that I should stay at home with my parents until the time came for me to move further into the system as my psychiatric deterioration became more manifest. For some reason, I refused to accept that prognosis. I knew deep down that I could get more out of life and I prayed frequently to God to help me to get that. Indeed, because I was fairly smart, I managed to get many positions in the security field which I would have been barred from had they done a background check on me. Such was the prejudice in those days against employing people with a mental illness record.

Of course, lots of people around me could not understand why in winter I was lethargic and in spring I would surpass everyone else's productivity. This was the seasonal edge to the many faces of the Ed Syndrome. However, although I often felt like someone with multiple personality disorder, beneath it all I had a sound set of morals and a keen sense of my inner strength. Both of these have helped me greatly in my recovery.

My attitude to a lot of the care that was offered me was certainly conditioned by my experience of my mother's treatment, especially the pharmaceutical lobotomy she and many others experienced, blunting rather than helping them. A lot of the doctors at that time kept patients and family members in the dark. I was therefore quite suspicious and dismissive of psychiatrists who just wanted to shove pills at me, without telling me what I might expect by way of side-effects, or what kind of life I might be able to lead under their influence. I was also suspicious of those who stuck narrowly to the medical model: those who stayed very much on the other side of that big mahogany desk, scribbling away on their pads and charts, scribbling the stock psychiatric answers to all those medical questions. It was then that my hackles would go up.

Experiences which weakened my defences led me to seek out more non-traditional people. They also led me to read a ton of books, from which I gleaned much help and guidance. Indeed, I got myself a physician's desk reference text and a DSM3 (*Diagnostic and Statistical Manual of the American Psychiatric Association*, 3rd edn), the psychiatrists' bible, to make sure that I knew as clearly as I could what might be going on, and what the psychiatrist might be making of all of this, and what they were not telling me about. Again, paradoxically, this poor treatment prompted me into a learning frame of mind. I had always been able to work up to that point, even if it meant drugging myself up to do so, though not with illicit drugs, mind you, but now I started to learn about my rights and entitlements and I also learned how to accept as well as seek help, rather than simply denying that I had those needs. The psychiatric system that had so damaged my mom and all her contemporaries was not going to do the same to me.

The weakness of the psychiatric system provoked me, like many of my co-consumers, to begin to develop my own means of support, both personal and interpersonal. This weakness also led, unwittingly, to the development of the consumer movement. I often look back to those early days and my early experiences of trying to be helpful to my fellow patients. I am reminded greatly of the good nurses I have met, those who had really mastered their skills. I think that I still carry that same sense of vocation to the teaching and the work I do in the field. They had a great effect on me and they remain some of my great role models.

It is important to acknowledge that serious mental illness such as I have experienced has had a devastating impact, not just on me but on those close to me. There have been times when I have become so depressed, when the paranoia and despair have dug so deep, when I have had the opportunity to end it all, since I have had easy access to the gun which I might use to blow my brains out.... I knew, however, that in killing myself I would also kill my father. I also knew, deep down, that I had something to contribute and that suicide would terminate any possibility of doing so. However, at times I did get preciously close to the edge.

As I have said, from early on I harboured ambitions of being the first socially conscious cop in my area; the first with a Bachelors degree in criminal justice. All the time I hoped that through a Masters I might rise high in the field. I could, indeed have been retired by now, at forty-seven. The illness clearly put paid to all of that. I often think about how my ambitions were blown away. However, what makes it easy is that I am not materialistic. All I have needed has been provided by my inner strength, by God, by my wife, who has provided for our material needs. We are now even looking to send our daughter to college and perhaps to move into a bigger home.

Unfortunately, one of the other impacts of manic depression is that people see me, and others like me, as unreliable and untrustworthy. This is not true of those who have got to know me, the real Ed, who give me all the respect that I am due, indeed all the respect that I need. I believe that, far from making me unreliable or untrustworthy, the illness has also given me the gift of compassion. I can see and feel the emotional pain of others and can respond creatively to help them. I respond not only as a fellow sufferer, but also as a person who is slowly learning the human skills that I have seen in the good psychiatric nurses and psychologists who have, in turn, been compassionate and caring with me.

My illness was devastating, obviously, for my family. I was always the stable, mature one, even from a very young age. I was, indeed, often the peacemaker when family strife was evident. When I began to be affected by my illness, there was no one to fulfil that role, which meant a very empty space in my family. My dad feared me, and my illness. Nonetheless, he was always there for me, always staying by my side. I take great comfort from the fact that before she died my mom could see that I was on my way to recovery from the illness which had so devastated her life.

I got involved with the consumer movement long before I made my career switch from security work, which had for so long been my only ambition. I got into the whole prosumer thing for quite common-sense reasons. I was cycling up and down. People saw me as not being dependable. When I was depressed I would practise avoidance. When I was up I would deal with any situation, no matter how challenging, much to everyone's amazement. I decided to take a big salary cut in order to take a job as an entry-level care worker at a psychosocial day-care centre not far from home, working with the seriously and persistently mentally ill. I augmented that work with evening security work, four or five hours on top of my full-time day job. Because I did not have my degree, I was relegated to more menial stuff – driving vans, recreational activities – which I grew to love. My supervisor was a rough type until he got to know me. I was still then in the closet, so to speak. I felt obliged to disclose my history and the agency director was initially very uncomfortable about letting the clients become aware of this. Eventually, however, I became respected and slowly moved to a new agency with greater responsibilities. I took on some case management work. I had just a small caseload initially, doing outreach work with people who were shut in with serious depression. I began to move into supported employment work, getting some training from the state *en route*. Although the whole self-help and support movement was growing, I was one of the very few people working in the field to have disclosed my own history of mental illness. Gradually, I began to be contacted by all sorts of other people who were in the closet but who felt that they too needed to come out and disclose their experience. Over time I began to be contacted by administrators, psychiatrists, psychologists, nurses, all sorts of people who were working in the field and who had also had experience of serious mental illness. Around that time I ran into the psychiatric nurse, Shirley Smoyak, who helped me greatly by opening all sorts of doors, helping me gain access to people and places both locally and nationally. Through the self-help clearing house at Philadelphia, I got involved with the national empowerment centre and met folks such as Dan Fisher, Judi Chamberlin and Pat Deegan. I began to present workshops on supported education, housing and my other experiences in the self-help field. The rest, as they say, is history.

I have learned a lot down the years, mostly about myself. Early on in my recovery, or growth process, like folks with an experience of physical illness or disability, I would seek condolences and pity. I was playing the 'poor me' syndrome without even realizing it. Of course, this served only to alienate and frustrate friends and family – indeed, all those who cared for me, including my wife. When I started to take a long, hard look at all of that, especially when I began to hear it in others, I think then I began to take the first step up that ladder of self-discovery. When I began to contrast my experience with that of others in the self-help movement, I began to see more clearly what was going on for me.

Through my illness I have become closer to God and my religion. I never developed an *unhealthy* approach to religion, although some do. I learned to equate in a biblical sense my illness and the suffering that God has promised us, both in the afterlife and here on earth. I equate my growth process with the search for the Holy Grail. I have gone through life running hither and thither in that search. Although I have got nowhere near finding the answer, I have learned a lot and have helped myself in the process, perhaps mainly by helping those around me. This may lie at the very heart of the recovery process. This may be the very nub of the idea of self-help, the ethic being that only through helping others can you help to heal yourself. I have met many fellow sufferers who eat, live and breathe the consumer movement. I have also met hundreds of professionals who similarly have committed themselves to the same ethic. And I have taken great strength from those who have made their own sacrifices to make their contribution. My search for the Holy Grail continues, but I do gain inner peace and inner strength along the way. At times I can lose sight of that and have to slow down, using some of those old yoga breathing techniques I learned, so long ago, from that psychiatric nurse. Sitting on the beach with that salt air hitting me in the face and seagulls swaying overhead, I can find the tranquillity that helps me look back on the good things I have experienced in my life; that helps me appreciate how the Grail is not to be found in this life; that helps me know that that will be OK, too.

There is still much that is discouraging. In particular, I struggle to work out why people cannot work together for a common goal. This is true of folks in the 'prosumer' movement as much as anywhere else, jockeying for position, making waves and generally getting into rivalry. It is true also in the fields of psychiatric, psychological and nursing education. Lots of the teachers are out of touch and are simply not teaching the right material. This is a great setback, when there is such a need for students to learn what makes people tick *in a human sense*. Even if people end up working in a highly medicalized area, it is vital that students recognize the importance of social, psychological and spiritual perspectives. This is, after all, what brought the patient into contact with the services in the first place.

I started to talk about myself as a 'prosumer' a few years back, and found out that other consumers were playing with the same concept (Manos, 1993). Acronyms, jargon and buzzwords clutter the world of discourse about mental health and illness. Knowing the meanings in this private vocabulary is a kind of ticket to the inner realm, or backstage, separating the informed from the ignorant; separating the insiders from the outsiders. 'Prosumer' is a neologism, born from a marriage of 'professional' and 'consumer'. A prosumer is a former pure consumer who has decided to look beyond self to the larger work to be done in the field. Funnily enough, blending consumer and professional in the proper sequential order would result in 'confessional'. That doesn't quite communicate what this new being is all about. Prosumers are former mental patients, graduates of various forms of living hell, transformed and activated toward a wide variety of work roles, focused on others who are still in the early stages of defining themselves and their beings.

Alvin Toffler, apparently, coined the word in his book *The Third Wave* (Toffler, 1980). Recently he has elaborated:

> Producer and consumer, divorced by the industrial revolution, are reunited in the cycle of wealth creation, with the customer contributing not just money, but market and design information vital for the production process. Buyer and supplier share data, information, and knowledge. Someday, customers may also push buttons that activate production processes. Consumer and producer fuse into a 'prosumer'. (Toffler, 1990:239)

In mental health services where folks have 'come out' about their experience of mental illness, prosumers can be particularly successful with patients and consumers who are still actively struggling with their illnesses, and who have not yet been able to develop good interpersonal relationships with their professional caregiver. People who have 'been there' can develop trust and show the way to new ideas and new ways of relating. The first steps are often simply toward accepting the illness. Not so simple, of course, but certainly rudimentary. We prosumers are more believable when we state that we have been there and know there is a way out. We are seasoned travellers. We are excellent guides. We know the ropes, we know the paths and we simply say 'Come follow me!'.

Once this early work is done, we are next very helpful in energizing folks who feel demoralized, weak, worn out and hopeless. For us prosumers, seeing a person gain new strength produces an absolute high, and gives us energy to work another day, put up with another insult, ignore ignorance.

Of course I am not so naive as not to know that some situations are simply too dangerous to do what I have suggested. Coming out and being honest about one's mental illness is still punished in many places. In such times and places, the work has to go on less openly. And finally the hard work, dedication and love will overcome the obstacles.

This takes me back to thoughts about love and obstacles in my own life. Although friends melt away with time, as I wrote earlier, true friends are still there for me. I still have one very good friend from early days, who has tried consistently to understand me and has taught me the value of true friendship. I need, of course, often to force myself to keep in touch with people, even when that is an uphill struggle. I need to keep working at the business of living and relating. But to make that easier, the prejudice against employing people with a mental illness record may be changing, albeit slowly. What is most important to me now is to take a step back from all of that, to do some real work on my family and my relationship to them. I need to get out on the two-man kayak which I bought this summer. I need to get out there with my son and try to become his friend as well as his father. I need also to put my wife in that same kayak and do much the same thing. She deserves no less. We married in 1976, and we are still going strong, more than twenty years down the line. I need also to find more of that inner peace and then use that peace to get back into the fray, all guns blazing. I will be aiming again for that important piece of paper that will help me get fully into teaching, although I would not want ever to leave the consumer movement behind me. It is important to keep involved, to keep touching the base, but I am keen to reach out to a broader audience.

I recall many years ago seeing a movie with James Stewart, called *The Flight of the Phoenix*. An aeroplane had crash-landed in the desert and the survivors had to salvage pieces of the wrecked plane. They would use these to make another plane, to give them the chance of survival. I relate strongly to the allegory of that film, echoing, as it does, so many aspects of my life where survival has depended so much on the way we salvage what we can from the wreckage. So many times I have been up, only to crash-land in my own desert. What I and many others in the consumer movement have discovered is that, given time, we can piece together a new life, which will help us find a new way out of that desert, rising like a phoenix from our own wreckage... if not from our own ashes.

References

Manos E (1993) Speaking out. Psychosocial Rehabilitation Journal 16 (4): 117–120.
Toffler A (1980) The Third Wave. New York: William Morrow.
Toffler A (1990) Powershift. New York: Bantam Books.

Chapter 6
Avalon

LIZ DAVIES

Editorial

The best view of the 1960s is from hindsight. From there we can pretend that it was all liberation and exaltation; all love, peace and responsibility-free hedonism. For most of the baby boomers the reality was quite different. Yes, there were new-found freedoms, but also many of the postwar restraints carried on in a more covert disguise. For young people, like Liz Davies, who caught the tide of idealism and cultural growth, the penalties of non-conformism could be great, although – of course – dispensed with her best interests at heart. The 1960s saw many young people reined in by the authority of psychiatry, simply because they had strayed from the well-trodden paths of their elders. The extent to which the benign paternalism of psychiatry has diminished in the subsequent 30 years is one of the issues upon which the reader will reflect.

Liz Davies was confronted by a pressure to conform. Actions that appeared to breach that boundary of conformity were interpreted as signs of mental instability. Her story is a powerful echo of Laing and Esterson's (1964) case vignettes from Sanity, Madness and the Family. *Her story illustrates the function of psychiatry as the long arm of society. At times, some psychiatrists wished that that arm could be even longer but, ultimately, one psychiatrist cut back his arm, affording Liz the opportunity to claim her own psychiatric rescue.*

Liz's story also illustrates the psychiatric 'catch 22' classically described by Joseph Heller. By owning up to her experiences Liz was condemned as mad and by denying them she was denying herself, and that way lies madness, anyway. In the vernacular, she was damned if she did, and damned if she didn't!

Liz Davies's story also reminds us of the power of natural community and, ultimately, of love. There was not, and perhaps still is not, much love expressed in the name of psychiatric care, but Liz finds it anyway in some of the relationships with her fellow travellers. Liz's tale may not be the story of ordinary madness, but may indeed be wholly extraordinary. The temporary insanity attributed to all who are temporarily derailed or who otherwise change their tracks belies the vision which may lie behind the derailment. Readers might reflect on the fragile nature of their own sanity in this respect, asking – in particular – where the 'madness' of their dream or visionary states connects with the sanity of waking consciousness.

If the reflections and responses offered by Liz and other contributors to this text are anything to go by, a system of mental health care based on a clear view of mental health, rooted in spiritual vision, rather than a medical model of the mind alone, would be a good starting place.

Reference

Laing RD, Esterson A (1964) Sanity, Madness and the Family. Harmondsworth: Penguin.

★   ★   ★   ★   ★

Introduction

I was fifty the other week, and went to the doctor to check that the medication I was taking for migraine headaches was not going to damage my health. Having read that Midrid is contraindicated if there is any suspicion of heart disease, I felt I should check that I was not causing my heart distress for the sake of some short-term head-pain palliative.

The local GP checked my blood pressure and assured me that at my age heart disease was most unlikely. She asked if the drug was helping the headaches. When I affirmed that it was, she prescribed me another 80. She asked how my son was progressing at medical school, and whether I had got my PhD yet. She was friendly, brusque and obviously busy – but I felt there was a good rapport between us, and I took the prescription, suppressing my vague niggling doubts. I was happy to let the possibility that I was damaging my heart be pushed aside by her no-nonsense approach.

As I took my prescription from her outstretched hands, and smiled my thanks, she looked down at my medical card and said in a rather interested voice, 'I see it says here you had schizophrenia when you were eighteen'.

My vulnerable heart constricted with the shock. I thought my whole connective tissue had collapsed inside, the structural edifice on which I built my social life just melted away. In a thin voice I heard myself say, 'That was a mistaken diagnosis. I'm absolutely horrified to find it's still on my medical record. You just can't imagine how awful that seems to me!'

'It says you were in hospital for three months. Well anyway, whatever they did for you, it worked, because you're fine now!'
'I was never ill!', I reiterated feebly. 'It was a mistaken diagnosis by the local GP. I was mixed up, certainly, and I could probably have used a good counsellor, but not ill, certainly not schizophrenic. I thought it was all behind me.'

As I started to explain to her what had happened, the tears welled up in my eyes and heart. I heard my voice telling her, 'The local GP had just done a crash course on recognizing signs of mental illness...'

She listened empathically, but I could tell she was in a rush to get to the next patient.

'Well, anyway, whatever they gave you it worked – because you're better now!'
In a flat voice I insisted, uselessly, in a last-ditch effort to enlist her support: 'But I was never ill. It was a mistaken diagnosis.'

I finally realized the hopelessness of explaining. I saw how it was easier for her to believe that I had suffered a disease I never had, than that a psychiatrist might have made a wrong diagnosis.

However, the tears were pouring down my cheeks at the memory of the iniquity I had suffered. She saw I was upset, and offered me a cup of tea. I accepted, thinking she was going to let me sit with her and talk through my experiences. But then she ushered me outside to sit with the receptionist and nurse. I declined the tea, and hastened off to walk away my sorrow unobserved, shaking off the slur and negative aspersions like a dog shakes muddy water from its fur. I would carry on as normal, going to work like a normal person, fulfilling my job as a University Laboratory Technician. But I could never truly regard myself as normal since my hospital experience. I was not, and never had been, a normal person. I knew that any show of normality was simply a necessary mask and masquerade.

I had not realized until now how close to the surface it all was, all the hurt and humiliation from that brief experience of compulsory hospitalization. Social annihilation overwhelmed me and my self-esteem plummeted suddenly as I stood before my doctor and re-experienced the full power of the total invalidation conferred by that diagnosis and my subsequent treatment. How could anyone ever take me seriously again? All my writing, my research, my ideas – all discredited, crazy! My research work (already in a much maligned and pioneering area of biophysics) could never be taken seriously, my work with emotionally disturbed teenagers, with people with learning disability, as a teacher with children in schools, and with healing groups, all this could never be taken seriously if it were known that I had this diagnosis on my medical record!

Thirty-two years had passed, yet I still bore the scar, with a wound as raw and fresh under the surface of its thin skin as on the day it was first inflicted. It had taken many years to plaster over this crack, and the knowledge that it had remained all this time in black and white on my medical record had stripped the plaster off in one fell swoop. Ouch!

Hubris

In 1965 one still talked of 'beatniks'. I identified with beatniks, in so far as I eschewed many social values. I walked the streets barefoot, slept in my clothes, wore home-made tunics of upholstery material held together by safety pins. Not all the time, however! I also wore normal clothes, including overalls to work in Sainsbury's, and boots and sandals in the vineyards and banana plantations of the Kibbutz. And I had worn normal clothes when I taught the children at Sunday School, after doing a year-long teacher training course throughout my first year A levels. I taught the children religion in a style different from my own much hated religious education. I used dance and drama and painting, and tried to get them to experience God in their little fingertips. My unorthodox methods, although encouraged by the leader of my training course, led to a sudden dismissal by the orthodox head of the synagogue school in which I was voluntarily teaching. This gave me my first great social invalidation experience.

In 1962 I had been asked to give a talk on mysticism at the local Young Socialist group headquarters. A friend of my cousin was investigating me as a 'mystic' after hearing about some of my ideas and practices and experiences. Indeed, many of the spiritual experiences I had by this time were echoed in the later psychedelia, specifically LSD experiences, of the 1970s. However, by contrast with the drug-induced mysticism that characterized the 1970s, my mysticism stemmed from hard internal questioning work, using intellectual focus and creative thinking, exercises in rajah yoga and meditation. This work led to a 'breakthrough'– an experience of enlightenment or realization about the nature of reality. It was an experiential realization of truth that is beyond conceptualization, and I recognized it as a point of no return. There was a fundamental change or transformation of my psyche, my brain cells and of my whole neuroendocrine system. It was an experience of great light and unity.

This experience was recognized and validated subsequently as an authentic mystical experience. It was recounted in *Studies In Religious Experience: Living the Questions* and *The Original Vision*, published by the Religious Experience Research Unit at Manchester College, Oxford.

I did not realize at the time that I was unusual in respect of the inner spiritual work I was undertaking. I did not realize that my friends were not pondering the origin and destiny and significance of the universe as I did, or gazing up at the night sky with such burning questioning, longing for a lost paradise.

I had been deemed a 'gifted' and creative pupil. I wrote and produced plays for my peers and for younger children, and participated in teaching younger children. Nevertheless, my teachers were very disconcerted by my ideas and by the despairing picture I painted, in my epic poems and plays, of a civilization whose values and standards I found spiritually repugnant. My sixth-form tutor tried to give me after-school counselling and reassure me that the adult world was not so bad. I told him it was worse than bad. We lived under the shadow of nuclear destruction.

Needless to say, my mysticism worried and frightened my parents. They found my ideas deeply disturbing, and my open rejection of some of their values hurtful and inconvenient. Nevertheless I was a kind and considerate daughter in many respects, even if a little crazy and rebellious, unworldly and idealistically naive. I was honest and hardworking, helpful in the home, and friendly and supportive to those around me (although often I must have seemed a little aloof and detached – I was deeply introverted). And I had been in love, since I was fourteen, with an artist, ten years older than myself, whom I had agreed to marry.

My fiancé had been brought up in an orphanage since the age of seven, after his mother died. My maternal instincts were aroused and I wanted to heal the motherless breach in him. Four years into our relationship, I discovered that his mother was in fact alive and in a mental hospital. She had been taken away when he was seven, and kept there ever since. He never saw her again; so she was 'dead' to him. My parents were very worried about this relationship, and had tried to discourage me from it.

I returned from a year's work on a kibbutz in Israel in 1965, during which time we lived together as man and wife. I intended to earn some money and prepare for our wedding while he completed his military service in Israel. I was not altogether happy about this, as I had missed my interview for medical school, and I was conflicted about how to reconcile marriage and career. My fiancé felt very threatened by my studying science, and actively discouraged me from pursuing it. Yet I knew I had some work to do in science, connected with healing and hidden fields. It has taken me thirty years finally to enter into that work as a PhD research scientist. But at that time I was confused and undecided about how to get there. I needed some positive help and support.

I threw myself into writing a children's book, and by the time I had completed two books in one month, my feet were three feet off the ground. I felt I needed grounding. I needed help to get to where I had to go. But I was exhausted from writing so intensively. I had a dream one night. In the dream I found myself:

> ...under the bowels of an ocean-going ship. The water is dark and murky, lit by an eerie phosphorescence, and I am lighting the fuse to blow the ship up. Hanging over the deck of the boat above me are the world destroyers, decadent people, world-haters and rejecters. A voice tells me suddenly that I don't have to blow myself up with them, I can take the right-hand side. Suddenly I look up and see a spiral staircase going up the right-hand side of the boat. I run up it as fast as I can, round and round, and when I get to the top, I burst out onto a platform, flooded with brilliant white light, on which stands a figure of a ballet dancer poised on a pedestal. I merge with the figure...

I took this dream to be a sign, literal rather than symbolic, that the study of dance would help balance and redirect my energy toward my life's goal. So the next day I took all my writing, got a lift with my father to London, and went in search of a recommended dancing teacher, to get grounded and begin to realize my dream.

I found the dancing teacher, but she was most unhelpful, and I realized I had got the wrong impression of her work and personality. She had a hair appointment and had to rush off. Foolishly I had not taken sufficient money for my return journey, so I went to my cousin's flat to await his return and borrow my train fare home. This was the start of an adventure that proved my downfall.

Nemesis

As I sat in the cold November wind and rain on the grey stone steps leading up to my cousin's flat, I was blissfully unaware that I was being observed from the house opposite by a plain-clothes detective, disguised as a gardener.

I waited and waited and got cold and stiff, and when a young West Indian appeared and invited me down into the basement to await my cousin's return, I gladly accepted and followed him down. Inside it was warm and steamy; there was a red and black sofa and a red and black drum set, there were some other men, talking and smoking, and beautiful children, from early teens to toddlers, running around. The children seemed too young and vulnerable to be motherless in a flat full of men and strangers. I wanted to care for them, and act as a bulwark against them and the crazy adult world. I followed the children round and found myself playing with the littlest one. As the afternoon passed, I helped cook for the children and later got them ready for bed. More people arrived, and I found myself sitting on the sofa next to an older West Indian man, with pale skin and greying hair. He had a saxophone with him. I asked him about the band that obviously rehearsed in the flat. I sang him some of the songs I had written.

'You like music? You write songs? That's good. We need another singer. Hey Jess, this lady could be our vocalist.'

I felt some measure of spiritual and emotional rapport with the saxophonist. He exuded a sort of weary wisdom. In addition, the idea of a white girl blending with a black scene fuelled my idealism; such amalgams might provide the fount of healing energy to create a world of racial harmony. I regarded this as divine opportunity, albeit mixed with its measure of future discomfort, difficulty and arduous endeavour. I was keen to learn and open to opportunity. I was naive and believed good of everyone.

Five minutes later, the door burst open and the room was filled with white men in grey suits. They tore the pictures off the wall, ordered us off the sofa, ripped apart cushions and chairs, overturned tables, swore and cursed at the West Indians.

'Who are you', I asked, 'And how dare you talk to these people like this?'

'We're plain clothes officers', they replied. 'We have a warrant to search these premises for dangerous drugs. What's a white girl like you doing in a place like this?'

I found myself standing up and heard my voice boom out over all the commotion: 'There are more dangerous things in the world than dangerous drugs. And the way in which you're treating these people epitomizes it. Wars are made of such hatred and disrespect for others.'

A policewoman shone a torch into my eyes.

'She's high as a kite.'

She was referring to my pupils, which were always enlarged, and she assumed this was a sign of my taking drugs.

'You'd better come to the police station with us, miss.'

'On what grounds? You have no grounds to detain me. I have nothing to do with drugs.'

'What are you doing here then?'

'I'm visiting my cousin who lives in the flat upstairs. I'm waiting for him to come back.'

They took my name and address. I agreed for them to ring my parents to confirm my story. They did, and of course unduly alarmed my parents.

'Don't worry, dad', I said. 'I'm not involved with any drugs. This is all a shock to me. I don't really know what's going on. I was just looking after some children living in the basement flat below Laurie, while I was waiting for him to come home. I didn't have enough money for my train fare. Then there was a police raid. The police are bullying these people and they're trying to take me to the police station. But I'm not going. I'll be home soon. Don't worry.'

My parents pleaded with me to go to my cousin straight away, which I did. I don't think the police found anything. But a glimpse I had caught when I first entered the flat of a gaunt and ghostly white lady, head down in some secret tête-à-tête with a plump West Indian gentleman in a side room, a dim red lamp and silver weighing scales between them, could have been, in retrospect, the negotiations of a heroin addict with her dealer.

Late that night, under the stars, my cousin lectured me about my parents' worry. He sounded so pompous, authoritarian and, like my father, reasonable, that the rebel in me surfaced. I refused to stay with him, but borrowed some money instead and told him to tell my father that I would return home in my own good time. Foolishly and rebelliously, I went with Mikey, the saxophone player, to stay in his rented room and learn about 'the struggle' I had unwittingly witnessed.

Mikey still suspected me for several days as an undercover police-woman and I felt trapped in a web of paranoia and deceit. So much for trust and racial harmony. Within five days, unable to wash properly or relax, I had contracted some infection. Mikey had wanted me to be his woman, and keep him warm all winter. He had helped me to find a job in a local department store. But I was sad and ill and disillusioned. I had to admit to myself and to him that I could not live with the paranoia and drabness of the London world he frequented. I invited him to come home with me.

'What would a black guy like me do in a middle-class white neigh-bourhood?', he said. 'Towns is vicious, man. They make a man develop mean and cunning.'

I sadly acknowledged the truth of it, and said goodbye.

More Nemesis

In the dismal carriage on the train, going home, I felt most unwell. I thought I was having a heart attack. An acute muscular spasm, like cramp, racked my whole chest cavity, so I could hardly breathe. The tears streamed from my face. For what seemed like ages, I felt in the grip of an iron claw, unable to move or speak. Eventually the pain abated a little, so by the time I reached my station, I was able to drag myself off home.

I thought I might be dying. But strangely I didn't mind, as prior to my one-week adventure in London, I had posed a mental question to my self:

'What shall I do?'
An almost immediate answer had surfaced from my unconscious self.
'Die!'

I was aware at the time that this probably referred to a spiritual 'death': the dying of 'self' or 'ego'; a state of transformation in which the old condi-tioned self is sloughed; a painful process accompanied by what mystics term 'The Dark Night of the Soul'. I didn't know how I might accomplish this, but the voice had alerted me to a radical transformation needed in my life, as though all the old ways and old energy patterns and plans needed to be discarded – were useless for whatever I had to do.

I was used to inspirational ideas, or an 'inner voice'. I had written poems under such inspirational guidance. One long essay, written under 'inspiration' as though it were dictated through me, was entitled 'The Mother'. This was a critique of society and its values, and the limitations of conditional love, epitomized in the conventional social role of the mother and the conceptual framework in which children are educated and indoctrinated into society. It was an appeal for a radical new education of children and a new social paradigm, in which the limitations of 'dearth' and 'division' would be replaced by an acknowledgement of bounty, unity and love. Amongst the opening words of the essay was the injunction: 'Kill the Mother'.

It was explained that this was not a literal physical death, but a deconditioning that would release the real spirit of the mother, a being of beauty and universal love.

My visit to the dancing teacher was an initial attempt to reorientate my life and find a new balance. I had set out on an adventure and, in a sense, relinquished some of my old control on my life. Now, with this sudden sickness and chest spasm, it suddenly occurred to me that perhaps physical death was on the cards. It seemed a radical way of transformation, but I had an open mind. Physical and metaphysical death were both possibilities. I was not afraid of death; I was fascinated by it. I had often pondered on the process, and even tried to hold my breath to see if I could approach or even cross the boundary, in order to understand what death was. It was an inevitable mystery, for which I wanted to be prepared. I saw it as a gateway to the fundamental level of reality and consciousness with which I longed to merge my being. Most of the time I felt trapped and cut off and confined in my human body, imprisoned in our existing social structure. I had hoped that dance as taught by this dance teacher might help to free my sense of limitation in the body and keep me happily grounded, although of course, as it turned out, my visit to her was ill-judged and ill-timed.

I can't remember whether I intimated to my mother that I thought I might have had a heart attack. Certainly, my mother was concerned that I seemed very ill, and so she called the doctor.

The doctor arrived. By now the pain in my chest had abated, but I was experiencing severe pain in my bladder and urinary tract. He asked me how I was feeling. I think I may have intimated that I thought I could be dying, but I really wasn't too concerned. This must have sounded very bizarre to him. But in my weakened, pain-racked state, I was not being careful what I said to him. I was opening my heart, revealing my whole psyche, naively and trustingly. I was not sufficiently aware of how my paradigm of consciousness and life was so alien and frightening to others. For a long time I had experienced and inhabited the world of myths, legends and archetypal forces. I was like a native in this territory, and spoke its language freely. Unfortunately I did not realize that others not only did not speak it, but wrongly interpreted it as a meaningless babble, a language of insanity and madness.

I told him about my writing and showed him one of my epic poems and its accompanying paintings, and talked about my dreams and visions for a new world, about the transformative role I longed to play, but didn't yet know how to.

He said, 'I've got a friend who would be very interested to meet you'.

My heart suddenly sank, and I knew intuitively that his 'friend' was a psychiatrist. I realized forlornly that I had been too open and indiscreet and inappropriately confiding.

'Is your friend a psychiatrist by any chance?', I asked bitterly.
'He is. I'm sure he'd like to meet you. Would you mind if I brought him round tomorrow?'

I was used to people showing interest in my poems and experiences. Some time previously my cousin had asked, similarly, if he could bring a friend round to meet me, as his friend was interested in mysticism and altered states of consciousness. This meeting had led to a long and rewarding friendship. So I said yes. And so it was that I opened myself to whatever fate decreed.

The next day the doctor arrived with his friend. The consultant psychiatrist was most bizarrely dressed in a black suit and black bow tie, and carried a black briefcase, although it was a Saturday and the sun was shining. He looked most out of place in a domestic setting, more dressed for a funeral than for an informal interview. The briefcase put me in mind of my cousin's friend when he had come round to interview me, so I was not too perturbed. He spoke to me for five minutes, and my parents for 20 minutes. During my interview he asked me 'Do you ever hear voices?'.

I wanted to answer honestly, without misleading him. I replied affirmatively, but moderated my reply: 'I listen to an inner voice. I know it's my own voice, but it's an inspirational voice.'

He hardly looked at me, but scribbled notes on a clipboard. After he had interviewed my parents, I found my mother weeping. I asked her what the matter was.

'Oh, darling. You're seriously ill. You've been ill for a number of years. If only I'd realized. If only I'd known.'

'What's wrong with me, mum?'

'You've got...' choked sobs almost obliterated the word, 'schizophrenia'.

The doctors and my parents told me I needed a rest. I agreed, although I resisted the idea of going anywhere at present, as I was in pain. The doctors became more specific. They told me a place was available in a very nice sanatorium, a cottage hospital in the country. The picture they painted appealed to me. It sounded quite romantic. I welcomed the thought of a quiet retreat for a few weeks in the country to get well and recollect myself. However, I saw no urgency, and said I would consider it. The doctor said I should go there at once, for my own good, and emphasized that if I didn't go voluntarily with my parents by car, that afternoon, they would instruct an ambulance to collect me at four o'clock. I was a little confused by this. Schizophrenia was an interesting label, but I didn't altogether understand the urgency surrounding it, and began to panic.

'What if I don't like it?'

'If you don't like it', they said, 'Of course you can leave the next day'.

I was badgered and cajoled by mum and dad. 'Do give it a try, dear', said my mother nervously. 'It'll be so much better if we all go there together in the car. I don't want an ambulance coming round to take you.'

I thought that, at the very least, it would be an interesting experience from which I could extricate myself if it proved not to be conducive to spiritual repair.

Ultimate Nemesis: the Therapeutic Regime

Later that evening, I found myself not in a chalet-style country sanatorium but walking into an enormous Victorian ward, with 20 beds on either side, harsh lighting overhead, women standing, shuffling, moaning, lying and ranting, and a smell of stale cabbage. I decided, suddenly, that this was not for me. It was all too familiar, and not at all the restful, idyllic country scene I had in mind. Fifteen months previous to this, I had worked in a geriatric ward of a large Victorian mental hospital, as an assistant nurse. The patients were mostly suffering from Alzheimer's, and the memory of the sadism and bullying of some staff, and of patient neglect, was still fresh in my mind. A cold horror gripped my heart, as I recognized this as an almost identical set-up. What had I foolishly allowed myself to comply with? Still, I had agreed to try it out, and I thought it could be interesting to experience a mental hospital from the other side of the counter, as a patient rather than a member of staff. One night was not too onerous, and it would give me plenty of fuel for writing. Next day, I determined, I would leave.

I was officially admitted that night by a young Indian psychiatrist, who asked my name and age, if I knew what date it was, and if I knew where I was. All these questions I answered correctly. I cannot remember anything else he asked me. But I was then shown to my bed, in the middle of the ward, at the end of one row, next to the toilets and sinks. I can't remember if there were curtains round the bed – I think not. I remember harsh lights interspersed with pools of darkness all along the dismal ward, and a lady in the bed next to me asleep, while another opposite me grumbled that she knew why they were angry with her, because she had left her shoes under the bed. A woman two beds up was tearing up a pinafore meticulously. Another woman stood in the middle of the ward, like a priestess, and proclaimed aloud, each word reverberantly staccato: 'Today ... I ... had ... a ... pear...;'

There was a long pause between each word, and now an even longer pause. Her face shone, intense.

'A ... peach...;'
She was in a state of ecstatic rapture.
'and ... now ... an ... apple!'

She continued to stand there, her hands clasped in a frozen act of amazing grace.

As in a dream, I remember getting into my nightie and hearing the screams of a woman who had put her fist through a window, and wanted to repeat the act, but was being given an injection to sedate her instead.

I dreamt that night that I was piloting a spaceship out into the middle of the Universe, beyond the milky way, with no way back. I was alone and destined to go on forever into this sea of stars and galaxies and cosmic dust, without ever arriving anywhere; no firm land, a lost soul. The terror of the emptiness and fullness of space evoked the recollection of my child-hood nightmares, an endless repeating pattern of white waves, the prelude to fever and blinding headache and sickness and despair.

I was awoken rudely by the light being switched on, and the rattle of teacups. I drank my hospital tea and determined to leave. I did not wish to experience any more of this living hell, this abyss of lost souls. I did not feel it was conducive to my physical well-being or spiritual repair. I was not up to savouring the experience. I decided to get dressed and leave at once.

I reached into my locker for my clothes. I couldn't find them. Where were my clothes? I asked a nurse. She was evasive. I went to find the sister, who explained to me that my clothes had been taken away. I did not need them at present, as doctor said I was to rest. I tried to explain to her that I had been told I could leave today if I didn't like it, and I didn't like it. I wanted to leave.

'Please give me my clothes.'
'I'm sorry, I can't do that. Go back to bed till doctor comes to see you.'
'When is the doctor coming?'
'I don't know. Tomorrow maybe.'

I felt I couldn't bear to stay that long. I tried to reason with the nurse, but to no avail. I had already conceded one night in this Kafkaesque fortress. I would be out of my mind to stay longer.

I felt like a trapped animal, and behaved accordingly. If I couldn't have my clothes to leave, I'd just have to leave without them. I realized with horror, though, that as things stood I would not now be leaving so much as escaping. Intuitively I realized I had been tricked and cheated into coming here. I was not free to leave at all.

I walked up to the glass doors at the end of the long corridor leading from the kitchens to the ward – the same corridor I had been brought along yesterday believing myself a free woman. The doctor's room led off to one side. The door was closed. Everyone was at breakfast, and unobserved I tried to open the main doors. To my shock, I found the doors were locked. I walked back and forward like a caged animal, my thoughts in disarray. I had to get out. Just then, the cleaning trolley came through the doors, and while the cleaner negotiated the corridor, I bolted through the swing doors in my nightie, and made for the woods outside, as in a living nightmare. The thoughts of how to hide and survive in a wood, as a drizzling rain was falling, flashed through my mind, but my first concern was to escape, wet or dry.

I heard shouts behind me and walked faster, not daring to look back. The shouts came nearer, and running footsteps were close behind me. I broke into a run; I had to get to the woods and hide, and wait for my captors to disperse. Then I could head for the main road and hitch a lift home.

Unfortunately, the nurses were faster than I was. Two of them grabbed me by the arms and linked their arms through mine. They were young girls, like me. I struggled a little.

'Let go! How dare you try to detain me.'

'I'm sorry, we can't let you leave just now.'

'Look at you in your nightie, soaking wet! What will doctor say?'

'Look, this is all a terrible mistake. I know you think I'm mad and so I haven't got a mind at all, but the doctor has made a big mistake. I'm just a poet. Put yourself in my shoes, a young girl who writes mystical poetry, full of ideals and revolutionary ideas. It's easy to misunderstand the language of poetry for the language of schizophrenia – but I'm not mad. I'm sane like you, and I want to go home.'

I begged and cajoled and reasoned, but to no avail. They were not young girls like me.

'We know, we know. You're getting all worked up and upset. You're not at all well, Elizabeth, and you need to rest and see the doctor. We're not allowed to let you run about like this.'

They goose-stepped me inside the building again.

'Now, are you going to stay in bed like a good girl, or do we have to give you an injection to calm you down? We can't have you running off like this again. What would your nice parents say?'

I was completely and utterly invalidated. Moreover, the nurses insisted I take some medicine and tablets the doctor had ordered – largactyl and stelazine. I did not want to, but when they threatened me with an injection, I complied.

'I demand to see the doctor!'

Each day I demanded, and waited, and no doctor appeared. I got angrier and angrier. Eventually I wrote a letter explaining my situation and gave it to the sister to give the doctor.

The medication made my mouth dry, my eyes light-sensitive and the world appear in monotone, grey and drab. It nauseated me and made me tired. All the sparkle of life had disappeared since I started taking the drugs they forced on me. I felt deeply depressed. I tried to avoid taking the medication. On one occasion, under the pretext of getting a drink, I dropped it into the water jug, which turned bright pink, and the nurse who followed me to make sure I swallowed it laughed and insisted I take another dose. On another occasion, I rushed into the toilets, on the pretext of getting a drink, and as I spat out the foul stuff, three nurses pounced on me and produced a syringe. They held me down on the floor of the toilets and threatened me with an injection if I didn't take my pills. Weeping, I

submitted and allowed myself to be poisoned orally rather than intra-
venously. It was less humiliating.

When eventually I saw a doctor, he asked me how I was feeling.

'I'm feeling awful', I said. 'I want to leave.'

He told me I could not leave until I was better. I asked him what was
wrong with me in his opinion. He told me I was detained under section 27
of the Mental Health Act, an order that committed me to psychiatric care
for at least 12 weeks. It had been signed by two doctors, and there was no
way I could leave. This information was entirely new to me and
confirmed that I had been tricked into complying. I told him that I had
been brought there under false pretences, and had been lied to by the
doctors who committed me. I told him the medication was harming me,
that it made me feel ill and depressed. I was sure it was damaging my
kidneys and liver, and that I might sustain long-term ill effects. (I was very
much into health foods and natural medicines.) I knew I had to stop
taking the drugs. However, the cold and supercilious Irish psychiatrist
had no intention of taking me off the drugs. As far as he could see, my
excitable behaviour and feeling awful were proof enough of my deeply
disturbed and psychotic state, and corroborated the excellent and correct
diagnosis of the other doctors. He told me that I needed the drugs to get
better.

'But there's nothing wrong with me, apart from this burning pain
in my bladder.'
'You're a very sick girl.'
'What do you think is wrong with me? ' I asked. 'I demand to
know what you consider wrong with me.'
'That's no concern of yours! You don't need to know.'
'But if I don't know what you think is wrong with me, how will I
know when I'm getting better?
'We'll know you're getting better when you recognize that you've
been ill.'
I angrily interrupted him: 'That's a Catch 22 situation! It's ridicu-
lous! Where's the truth in it? You're assuming that you're right
about my being ill and I'm wrong.'
'You're a very rude little girl – don't interrupt!'

It was some time before they treated my real illness. It was discovered that I
had been suffering from a severe attack of cystitis, which, the nurse told

me, could easily have initiated the chest pain and muscle cramps I had experienced.

'Pain radiates', she said.

It took a long time to clear, as a result of the staff's choice to treat my healthy mind, and ignore my sick body. I'm surprised I didn't suffer kidney damage.

Out of all the humiliations, the most damaging was the forced medication. On one momentous occasion I was given stelazine without the antidote. This caused a horrendous pressure in my head, and left me with a feeling of impending doom and dimming of consciousness which lasted for several hours, followed by an unrelenting spasm of neck and facial muscles, so that my head contorted continuously, turning almost by 90 degrees, and attempting to continue to 180 degrees. I was in agony and abject terror for hours, as I did not know the cause. The charge nurse told me sternly that I had probably brought it on myself by doing yoga exercises. The thought that I had unwittingly and foolishly damaged my neuroendocrine system made me feel truly suicidal. I felt worse than insane, I felt hopeless.

I believed my body to be a wonderful gift donated to me for life for the purpose of helping to heal the sick world. But if the healer was only capable of inflicting wounds on herself, what hope was there for the world?

My parents came to visit and, seeing my misery, begged the sister to do something for me – to call a doctor. The sister had to give me an injection to put me to sleep, out of my contorted misery. It seemed as though I was in the throes of one enormous unremitting epileptic fit, without loss of consciousness. My parents had to watch helplessly while I suffered.

Only later the following day did another nursing sister tell me the truth – that the devastating seizure I had experienced was the fault of the nursing staff, who had forgotten to give me the antidote. This knowledge caused me considerable relief, and I was very grateful for the honesty of the sister. It reassured me that it was not my fault. Needless to say I also felt very angry at the negligence and deception, and, more than ever, felt it imperative to discontinue this medication and leave the hospital. However, the angrier and more expressive I got, the more they dismissed my pleas as signs of madness. I wrote letters and asked for interviews, but to no avail.

Other patients counselled me to take the medication and, when the doctors asked how I was feeling, to say: 'Much better, thank you.'

By complying with the treatment I stood a chance of getting out. By resisting, I never would. The horror of my situation and the wisdom of their advice sank home, and I revised my strategy.

In later years, I realized that my enforced and unnecessary treatment had much in common with the psychiatric treatment meted out to Russian dissidents during the communist regime. I now believe I might even have been able to claim compensation, had I taken up my case with a good lawyer. Even if it were difficult to negate the official diagnosis, it might at least have been possible to establish wrongful administration of medication in this instance. Unfortunately my family were so much in awe of doctors that they preferred to turn their anger inward, rather than fight. This made me very angry with them. I remember calling them 'worms' and 'cowards' in their uncritical deference to black-jacketed, briefcase-carrying, white-coated, stethoscope-holding 'gods'.

When I expressed my anger at the damage the treatment was doing to me to another more senior consultant, he pleaded kindly: 'We're only trying to help you to sort out your life, you know, Elizabeth.'

He was grandfatherly and seemed upset that I should misconstrue the motives of the medical elders.

'Far from helping me sort out my life, you're actively making many difficulties.'
'What do you mean?'
'Well, for example – I was intending to get married. My fiancé was coming back from Israel in the Spring. But his mother has been in a mental hospital all his life – and he told me that she was dead to him. Now he's heard I'm in a mental hospital, what will he think? I will be dead to him, and he won't come back. I know it. I haven't heard a word from him since I was committed. So, far from helping, you're actively hindering my life.'

The rejection by my fiancé was real. I never heard from him again; at least, not until the day of my wedding to another man. This caused me great anguish. I understood its cause, but suffered deeply.

It was not only this aspect of 'sorting out my life' that was being sabotaged by compulsory hospitalization. It was also my whole self-confidence. Although I believe the experience fundamentally strengthened my belief in my real self and real value and stripped me of pretensions and worldly aspirations, it ill prepared me for fitting into the conventional social world as an adult. In many ways I'm glad about this. I have retained an independence and youthful or child-like quality that renders me immune to many adult distractions and social games. But it also leaves me feeling an outsider. I find it difficult to compete, feeling as much a loser as a winner. I recognize my own gifts and value, but don't expect anyone else to. Experience has taught me that my real value is often unrecognized and misconstrued by others. And I often wonder if I actually have any extrinsic value. This constant questioning of my extrinsic value makes me a poor candidate for competition and often I actively avoid it.

My ability to maintain my sense of an integral self throughout this episode was helped by an already flexible and integrated psyche, by yogic exercises, by a writer's sense of humour and pathos, by actively entering into relationships and dialogue with many other patients, and by crocheting a multicoloured magic blanket for my much loved youngest brother, one of the editors of this book. Ben still has this blanket, and still believes in its magic qualities! It certainly helped me to keep sane and calm and to protect myself in an aura of light and colour – very necessary, as the medication seemed to undermine those very healing qualities of consciousness.

The sense of personal suffering was made more bearable by identifying the process I was undergoing with a more archetypal suffering, a process of cosmic significance that put my own crisis into perspective.

The Priest-king

During this first month's incarceration, I began remodelling a play I had started writing while in Israel, entitled 'The King'. This story featured a main character, a king, who was suffering from 'schizophrenia'. He was split into two parts, one the *Player King*, a political agonist, engaged reluctantly in the struggles of maintaining the confidence of a disintegrating Kingdom, and the other a recluse, poet and dreamer, who would sit before a cave, contemplating the sea and refusing to engage with the world, a *Shadow King*. The two characters would occasionally coincide and speak simultaneously, in a poetic duo, at moments of key dramatic and emotional intensity.

The Shadow King, as he was depicted in the play, had a strong significance for me. During my adolescence, not only was I something of a recluse, poet and dreamer, as described earlier, but I also had a driving urge to live in a cave overlooking the sea. I could see this cave in my mind. I imagined the long cream-coloured woollen robe that I would wear in this cave. I worried about how to keep warm and dry and light a fire without matches. At the end of my hospitalization, and for many years after, I had dreams that I was flying like a bird over the west coast of Scotland, looking down on deserted islands, wild and remote, looking for my home, looking for a cave. I could see the islands clearly as I hovered over each one, sometimes zooming in for a close-up, so I could hear and see the sea pounding and crashing on the rocks.

I subsequently found my cave. In fact, I'm writing this now on an island known as Holy Isle, where my longed-for cave existed, overlooking the sea. The story of my search for this cave, also the story of the many others who are utilizing the power of this island and the cave for healing, seems relevant to the request I had recently to write my story. It is very difficult to write about these experiences, and at first I was inclined to turn down the request. I'd much rather forget this episode of my life. But while on the island, I listened to stories of some who had suffered from poor psychiatric treatment. This encouraged me to think that my story could be useful and relevant to a reappraisal of the treatment regime in hospitals, and an understanding of the needs of healing of different mental states.

The story begins some years ago, though. In 1945, my father was based on a minesweeper off the coast of Arran, a small island off the Firth of Clyde, on the west coast of Scotland. He was involved in naval exercises during the last stages of the war, and he had rented Sea View Cottage in Arran's main village, Lamlash, for my mother, an idyllic refuge from the devastations of the blitz in London. My parents remember their sojourn on Arran with great fondness. It was on Arran that I was conceived. Although I don't believe my parents ever took the boat trip across the small stretch of water to Holy Isle, nestling just off Arran's coast, I would first have 'seen' Holy Isle through my mother's eyes and from the safe confines of her womb.

In 1984 I made a return pilgrimage with my son to Arran. We took a boat ride from Lamlash to Holy Isle and, although at that time I had not heard of Holy Island, I recognized at once the spiritual sanctuary I had been seeing in my dreams. Saint Molaise's cave evoked a deep sense of connection with my mother's Irish Catholic roots and all the deep mystery of this spiritual heritage.

It was also in the mid-1980s that my youngest brother became a Buddhist. My mother had lamented, 'Why can't he do something sensible with his life?'. My response was, 'What could be more sensible than following a spiritual path?'

'He could join the BBC', my mother had suggested.

However, I agreed to investigate the organization and attend meditation classes to check the integrity of the teaching. I became impressed with the way in which this Buddhist group was disseminating sound spiritual teachings in a relevant, modern way. I came to see a fundamental connectedness in the roots of Judaism, Christianity and Buddhism, especially in the contemplative practices and in the ethical teachings which involve in all three the forgiveness of enemies and the love of one's neighbour as oneself. I reassured my mother that the Buddhist pathway was a safe one.

In 1990 I began to attend meditation classes with this same Buddhist group in an old vicarage that had once been my home, along with my husband and my son. And it was in 1992 that I read in a newspaper that Holy Isle was being purchased by Tibetan Buddhists as a retreat centre. I felt a sense of joy and relief, as if my life had come full circle at last. Soon after reading this article I came across a leaflet in a Brighton bookshop, inviting members of the public to participate in the Holy Island Project, specifically in early conservation work under the auspices of the Scottish Conservation Group in alliance with Samye Ling, the Tibetan Buddhist Centre that had now purchased the island, under the direction of Lama Yeshe Losal. I decided I wanted to be involved at the outset of this new stage in the history of Holy island.

My son and I drove up to Arran from Sussex on 22 July 1992, for a week's voluntary conservation work on Holy Isle. We didn't know what to expect, as we had had no personal connection with Samye Ling and knew no one. We only knew that everyone there would be volunteers and living conditions were primitive. We had brought tents, and our brief was to help in the construction of a dry-stone wall, in rhododendron control and in beach clearing.

We were relieved and gladdened by our warm welcome to the island, and by the industrious and intelligent community of a dozen or so people assembled there by Colin Moore, co-ordinator of the project. There were people from all walks of life: a Buddhist monk, a civil servant, teachers, social and community workers, a writer, a musician, an ecologist, a cleaner, a forester, a secretary. Many of the group had no previous connection with Samye Ling Tibetan Centre or with Buddhism, but had been drawn by the nature of the project. We followed an almost monastic routine, rising at 6 am to the sound of a gong for a period of optional meditation, followed by breakfast, then work until lunchtime at 12.30 pm and rest until 2.00 pm followed by a further work period until 6.00 pm. The construction of the dry-stone wall around the proposed vegetable garden was being supervised by Andy, a talented young university graduate and founder of an active student Scottish Conservation Group. I sincerely hope that the few foundation stones successfully laid by my son and me will still be there in 30 years time! I encouraged myself during this painstaking toil by thinking of the parable of the man who built his house on stone. Some of the rejected stones had a suspiciously sandy texture.

One of the outstanding features to me of Holy Island was St Molaise's cave, and I made a visit to the shrine at the earliest opportunity. I found it occupied by Sophie, a young woman in her thirties, and the third member of the resident caretaking community. Sophie, a museum curator from Belgium, had been living in the cave for two weeks, meditating and praying for ten hours a day, at least. When she saw me approaching, she invited me in without speaking, beckoning me to join her on the wooden bench, and offering me tea from a flask, freshly brewed with water from the healing spring next to the cave. I gladly accepted and stepped down into the cave. We sat looking out at the sky and gulls through the long slit of a window-like opening and listening to the sound of the sea pounding below. It was clear from the joy and lucidity in Sophie's eyes that the healing power of the cave had wrought some inner magic in her, which she later openly professed to be true. I was deeply moved and touched, as I felt the cave had come to life since my last visit more than eight years ago, and was being used as it had been in ancient times by St Molaise, as a place of prayer and healing. I looked around at the shrine containing both a simple wooden cross and an image of the Buddha. Driftwood was neatly piled by the hearth fireplace used by the Celtic saint in the fifth century, and there was a wooden bench, built by Sophie from a plank of driftwood and mounted on stones, containing a small pile of spiritual books, an alarm clock and candles. A mattress, neatly folded with a sleeping bag in the corner, testified to the sum total of Sophie's creature comforts in the cave, and a bowl of fruit in an alcove bore witness to the food offerings brought by visitors to the cave, as a token of care for her sustenance during the retreat.

How wonderful, I thought, that in our modern age, a young woman can safely, in the age-old fashion, undertake a spiritual retreat in the simplicity of a holy cave, and instead of being assigned to the nearest mental asylum, be protected and catered for and nurtured by a spiritual community during her sojourn. Two profound asthma sufferers on the island, Sophie herself and Jan, a volunteer, had been free of all symptoms since they first set foot on the island. Many years ago, in hospital, Sophie had actually died during an asthma attack, and was revived only by extensive resuscitation techniques. Holy Isle, she said, was the only place she had ever been able to live without asthma. She had been there for five months already.

I thought how easily national and religious intolerance engenders wars, but how the fruits of all true spiritual experience are love, peace and healing. The Tibetan Buddhists, like the contemplative Christian orders, encourage the experience of spiritual truth, which is beyond the definition of any one religion. Any place on earth that can help to encourage the 'love of the living God in the heart of man', as promised in Deuteronomy, must be of great significance today. Such, I believe, is the role of Holy Island.

The compassionate side of Buddhist spiritual discipline is epitomized in the Lothlorien community, another centre set up by the Samye Ling community, which caters specifically for people undergoing personal crisis and mental breakdown. This Scandinavian log-cabin-style building, in another location in Scotland, functions as a separate counselling retreat centre. It is a tribute to the fundamental teachings of goodwill and compassion in Buddhism that they are able to both preserve their own integrity, and at the same time share their discipline with the often confused and alienated Westerners who come to them for spiritual renewal.

I left Holy Island with a sense of some deeper underlying spiritual purpose to this alliance between ancient Christianity and Tibetan Buddhist teachings, and great faith that the group at Samye Ling would revive the full spiritual healing heritage of Holy Island within the next decade, and I also felt a deep connection within myself to the history of the holy cave.

St Molaise (otherwise known as St Laisren) was born to the Royal House of Ulster, in Ireland, and showed gifts of healing from the age of 3. He lived in the cave on Holy Isle for more than 30 years, acting as healer and counsellor to the people of Arran, and was an associate of St Columba. When his father died, his mother urged him to come back to Ireland and become King of Ulster, but he refused, and obtained permission from the Pope to continue his ministry on Holy Island. His story, unknown to me at the time of writing my play 'The King', bears an uncanny resemblance to my character of the Shadow King.

At the time of writing it is 1996, and this year on Holy Island I spoke in depth to three people who had experienced psychotic breakdowns as the result of drugs: in two cases marijuana, and in the other case LSD. A young man, in his first-year geology course at university, was introduced to hashish at a party. He had a bad reaction to the drug, which sounded to me like a complete poisoning of his system, leading to 'psychosis'. One man's meat is another man's poison, as the old saying goes, which seems to be true of drugs, both legal and illegal! He was treated in a mental hospital with more 'anti-psychotic' drugs. Not until his mother got him a place in the Lothlorien community did he feel that he received the help he needed. The Lothlorien community is run as a total environment, with an equal ratio of staff to clients. It seems he was able to talk and relate to others without being pathologized. He was listened to, not drugged, and allowed to heal himself.

A forty-year-old man, who had been labelled 'psychotic' throughout his life from late teens onwards, having taken LSD, was enabled to discontinue the medication he felt was making him ill, by following an ordered and spiritual life within the Samye Ling community. And a 50-year-old retired teacher described the frightening and counter-productive treatment she had been exposed to in a mental hospital, which increased her sense of paranoia, after 'friends' had cajoled her into taking pure marijuana extract to which she had reacted very badly. Two years later she was still suffering from the ill-effects. She had been told she had had a 'psychotic' breakdown. Again, this breakdown was caused by drugs that alter perceptual awareness and affect the neuroendocrine system. The further use of drugs was counter-productive. Other patients urged her to comply with the treatment in order to get out quickly.

I had been forced to take drugs myself, as a patient, never having taken any psychoactive drugs before. The drugs were wrongly administered on at least one occasion, making me feel out of control and very ill. I maintain that had I not been sane and healthy already, this treatment regime itself could have caused me to have a severe nervous or psychotic breakdown. If I had truly been suffering from schizophrenia, the treatment I received could have permanently damaged my health, both physical and mental.

So I am writing this, having started it on Holy Island, in the hope that 'treatment' of mental illness will be modulated to include 'understanding' and 'listening' in many cases where the diagnosis of 'psychosis' may be made appropriately, and 'discernment' where it may not. And that those engaged in healing mental confusion will develop a deeper understanding of mental coherence and the language of higher, altered, integrative states of consciousness so as to discern between a psychotic and a seer. We live in an age of conditioned, repetitive, fragmented, derivative and unoriginal thinking. Is it any wonder that originality is mistaken for 'disorder'? It stands out like a sore thumb and the dull and tidy-minded find it threatening or challenging.

The Firebird Flies Free at Last

However, back to the hospital ward, for the finale to my three-month episode. I had already been there one month, and I received a letter from my school friend, Jennie, who, unlike me, had agreed to sit the Oxbridge entrance exams and was now studying English at Oxford, to the delight of her parents. My parents would have liked me to do the same. But I knew that the study of English Literature was not for me. I had to master science.

Dear Liz, my tutor has a friend who knows what you are doing. She understands the sort of spiritual things you are into and she says you are in great danger. If you can, come to Oxford; she will be able to advise you.

I wondered what sort of danger she could mean.... I was not into Voodoo, or Ouija boards, or spiritualism of any sort. Her concern and invitation made me feel restless. I was getting no real-life counselling or spiritual guidance in the hospital. It felt as if life was passing me by, and I was trapped in a time-warp. Although I had started playing a game of co-operation in order to hasten my release, I knew it was a game, and that the whole situation was actually very wrong and dangerous. It was a game I did not want to play, but now I had no choice. My own folly had forced me to play it, and I had no idea how long the game would last. This breath of fresh air from the outside world made me feel impatient and restless for a change of scene.

I was allowed to walk around the grounds and visit other patients in other wards by now – a token for my good behaviour and 'progress'. A young male patient had befriended me. He was a doctor's son who had tried to kill himself. He suffered from depression, and was very cynical and bitter. We used to sit for hours in the grounds, talking, or walking in the snow. Recently he had left, promising to return with his father to rescue me, but nothing had happened, and I missed his company.

One morning, I just gathered up my purse and crochet in a bag, and walked out through the grounds and caught a bus, and then a train to Oxford, arriving at my schoolfriend's flat as dusk was falling. I was pleased with myself for having found the place so effortlessly – it was the first time I had visited her there. She was delighted to see me and chatted away, telling me her news and how it was at Oxford: her drama club, her boyfriends, her tutors and assignments, and how she had been to Israel recently and called in to see me on the Kibbutz, unaware that I had already left. My fiancé was there on home leave from the army, and he was missing me, so she'd slept with him that night as consolation. This piece of news disturbed me somewhat, and I looked at her anew, wondering just how much of a friend she really was.

She suggested we went out to supper. The Oxford scene felt exciting after being incarcerated for four weeks, and I gladly accompanied her, marvelling at her latest transformation from chic sophisticate to robust student, in a navy donkey jacket and short skirt. The Jennie I was used to wore her mother's mohair coats and designer clothes from Harrods. She seemed a little different, less sure of herself now she had left home and left her parents' world behind.

The phone rang, and she answered.

'Yes, she's here.'

My heart sank. It seemed her parents had been contacted by the police, who were looking for me. I hadn't realized how famous I was, and how important. I couldn't believe that so many people were going to so much trouble on my behalf. I didn't want my whereabouts to be revealed. I had only just arrived; I wanted to be free and anonymous. But Jennie was acting responsibly. It seems the police had contacted her tutor, and the tutor duly appeared on the scene, with a tweed-jacketed arm to put around poor Jennie's shoulder to console her, while her desperately ill friend was removed from her flat by uniformed police and hospital staff.

I was taken to a local psychiatric hospital where the nurses put me to bed and forced me to take sleeping pills – something I had never done before. I was terrified, but somehow resigned myself to the inevitability of this dehumanizing treatment. When you are at rock bottom, you can't get much lower. The fight in me was changing to a quiet detachment. I had been so deeply disillusioned and shocked by so many things recently; my new understanding of the world and human nature was causing me to reassess my reactions to it. Fight and flight were obviously counterproductive.

The next morning, I was invited to participate in a group-therapy session. The whole working of this ward was radically different from the ward I was used to. Patients here had jobs to do. It seems they swept and tidied as though they owned their own environment. The staff sat in an informal circle with the patients, and I was introduced as 'a young schizophrenic with suicidal tendencies from Netherne Hospital'.

This was the first time I had heard my official diagnosis read to me by medical staff. Now I understood why the police were called out, and why they were at such pains to detain me: they thought I might kill myself. How ironic that the treatment I was receiving was the only thing that had ever made me want to kill myself. I wonder how I survived it. If I had been really suicidal, my 'treatment' might well have succeeded in pushing me over the edge.

I met other patients and heard their stories of alcoholism and abuse, of violence, of mania, depression and suicide attempts. I discovered that they had a patients' newsletter and charter, and some sort of organized voice for representation and complaints. They advised me to write my story, and suggested that there might be some committee where I could have my case reviewed and reassessed. I felt a glimmering of hope. But this was quickly extinguished.

I seem to remember a long journey back in an ambulance. It was all so humiliating. I felt such a non-person, treated condescendingly by staff and doctors, discredited. I was no longer taken seriously. I had no hope of being fairly heard or represented any more. It is as if no one could see beyond the label of my madness or illness now. I was lost, labelled and destroyed.

Back at Netherne, we were allowed to earn three shillings and sixpence a week doing occupational therapy, which involved sewing electric blankets on a machine. It made a change. I got to speak to other patients from other wards. One tall, gangly young man told me how he had been ruined by doing spiritual exercises to raise the kundalini energy. He had raised it too soon and it had burnt through all his nervous system. He was left feeling as though he were on fire, and had been ill ever since. I knew from my reading what he was talking about, having read of an Indian holy man who had gone through just such a forced opening of the chakras when his body was not in a fit state to adjust to the energy. It had taken years of patient nursing by his wife, and a very special diet, to bring him back to normal functioning. But obviously the hospital did not understand this, and merely labelled this condition as 'psychosis'. I felt worried and concerned for this young man, but could only sympathize. The occupational therapist looked a kind and imaginative woman; she was Spanish. One day she gave me some motherly advice:

> You shouldn't be in a place like this, a girl of your age. When you get out, you make sure you behave yourself, and don't come back!

Suddenly I felt like a naughty schoolgirl who was being punished. This hospital was my prison. This view was confirmed later, when an older psychiatrist was summoned to assess me for possible psychotherapy. While he listened to my story his grey moustache bristled and his eyes narrowed.

'You're a selfish girl', he said. His voice was bitter with dislike.
'You hurt everyone around you, and you always will...!'

So much for dreams of healing the world. My shrink had caused my dreams to shrivel. Far from being a healing balm, he said I was an active harm. His callousness shook me, and I had to see his reaction to me as based on his own hurt as a father or grandfather, whose children were rebelling and rejecting his values. So much for objective assessment and empathy!

Later, another young psychotherapist to whom I was assigned listened while I attempted to bare my soul. He acknowledged, suggestively, that were we to meet on board a ship he would be fascinated and enticed by my seduction. But he was here to be my therapist. Whereupon he changed the position of our chairs so that our knees were touching. I was most confused.

Not only was I being invalidated in terms of my mental integrity, but my ethical integrity was also being denied and challenged. My sense of self-worth was utterly confounded.

As I ceased to struggle, a calm descended on me. It was Christmas, and part of the ward was being removed to a house in the grounds, a more homely and intimate unit. This seemed to encompass a number of the younger patients, including me. So, from being in a long open ward, reminiscent of the geriatric unit, I was now in an upstairs bedroom, smaller and square, with five other patients. I had a window next to my bed overlooking the grounds, and beyond them the trees and fields and hills. Downstairs was a dayroom with a Christmas tree, and a table on which I felt I could begin a daily routine of writing. I decided to occupy my time creatively in copying out and illustrating the children's stories I had written for my youngest brother. This helped me to keep calm, and a sense of timeless inevitability enfolded me. I even felt as if I could happily continue here forever, writing and dreaming. I no longer felt involved with the outside world. I no longer wanted to be or to do anything.

I met Freddie, a young West Indian with an Oxford accent, who was convinced that when he was in his 'glory' I would see him as he really was: white skin, blond hair, blue eyes. He said he would come for me next week and create for me seven universes of exquisite beauty. He would be God, the father, and I would be his secretary. He had no backs to his shoes. We sat in the graveyard and talked of heaven. Freddie told me he was wearing two pairs of swimming trunks, and when I asked him why, he said it was so I could not see his erection. We walked round the nearby caravan site commenting on the ephemerality of the world, its edifices and aspirations. We had tea in a local teashop with a lady who could not stop the convulsions of her head and mouth, or the trembling of her hands, that resulted from the drugs she was taking. We even went to the cinema. Our exploits took us further and further afield. And one day I took Freddie home to meet my mother, but when she saw his blackness, she shut herself in the bathroom and refused to emerge. We had to leave and return to the asylum without a welcome.

Freddie's insanity made me feel at home and befriended. The world of the insane began to feel kinder and more natural to me then the world of the sane. Constance, an actress, was sharing my dormitory. She was incarcerated for stabbing her husband. We had some good fiery talks. She said to me, 'Whatever you do, don't get like her!' pointing to Janet, a 25-year-old house-wife who stayed in her dressing gown all day and was suffering from a deep, almost catatonic depression. 'Nothing coming in, nothing going out! You want to have lots going in and lots coming out. Me, I'm the sort of person when I'm at home who pulls the chain at least five times a day!'

I said I thought that at least Janet was expressing her sadness and not covering it up and pretending to be bright. Anne, a heroin addict, who was deeply depressed but got up daily and dressed smartly and put lipstick on, got very upset and angry with me. She felt I was getting at her. Constance, who also made an effort to dress smartly, with new outfits every day and make-up and nail polish, got furious, and slapped me round the face. Later she apologized. But I understood. Truth was painful. *Get-up-and-go* was a camouflage, a way of coping with the pain.

There was an anorexic girl on the verge of death, and a pathological liar who got me to break into a house with her on the pretext that it was her house, and her husband had locked her out. Psychopaths, paranoid schizo-phrenics... we all had our labels. One woman had set fire to the ward; she used to be a nurse herself. She was beautiful and glamorous, and her husband was a wealthy businessman who visited her regularly in his ermine-collared wool coat. Yvonne crocheted herself the most beautiful feminine pink chemises, laced with pearls and silk. She wore an expensive fur coat and hat with a muff, but she wanted to burn herself alive. One day she set fire to her bed while she was in it.

There were warm people and cold people, lucid and crazy people. But the best therapy we ever had was from each other and our own play-acting. One night I instigated a role-play of our madness and we jumped on the beds and proclaimed 'This is an asylum and we're mad women'. We objecti-fied our madness and made fun of it, also making a mockery of the staff who were so terrified of accepting it. The only interaction we had with nursing staff was through pills, food and ECT. Very few patients got to talk to a doctor more than once a week, and then only for a few minutes. Constance had not seen a doctor for ages. I remember one white woman from Barbados, who was weeping and shivering with fear at the treatment they were going to give her that morning. That was the first time I had heard of ECT and of its adverse effects. It caused considerable pain, apparently, and caused burns and unbearable muscle spasms. I had heard about another patient in the open ward who slept all day opposite me. She had been given insulin coma therapy, followed by ECT, to alleviate deep depression after childbirth. It had worked temporarily, shaking her out of catatonia. But then she regressed and got slower and slower, and stood by her bed, shaking her head sadly at nothing at all. I found it difficult to understand how such a treatment as ECT could be of benefit, when it caused such distress and had to be repeated time and time again. I was very glad I did not have to suffer this treatment. It seemed there was no choice. Once you were diagnosed schizophrenic, your rights to consultation or decision or privacy, and your control over your own body, were taken away from you. A patient's human rights were denied once the label of schizophrenia was plastered on. Forced feeding, forced medication, forced hospitalization, forced ECT, total invalidation was the order of the day, once two doctors had signed a certificate declaring the patient to be suffering from schizophrenia.

Into this new, more liberal and intimate regime a new element was introduced: 'Group Therapy'. A number of us were chosen to be part of a pilot group. We sat in a room for a quarter of an hour in silence, until a patient suddenly blurted out: 'Isn't anyone going to say anything?'

'How do we feel about the silence?', asked the therapist. 'Doesn't it make us all feel uncomfortable.'

It was the first time I heard other patients describe their illness, and understood what a nervous breakdown was. It made me realize with certainty that I had never been ill like some of the women there, who really needed help to put themselves together again. Patients described to me their paranoid delusions, and how they affected their lives, and how they were relieved and glad to have help.

We also had an exercise and relaxation class in the dayroom, which I enjoyed. Blankets were provided on the floor, and our bodies were being honoured at last with a treatment of normality, a healthy dose of stretching, comfort and repose, and someone with a voice that seemed to care about each of us individually. This was something designed to make us feel better, to aid our well-being. It felt caring and good. I was grateful.

I remember only one interaction with nursing staff that was meaningful. A young Mauritian nurse caught me staring wistfully out of the window and came to talk to me, not as a patient but as another human being, another young girl like herself. She talked about her homesickness and asked me how I was feeling. I felt a kindred spirit, a real contact. Her own loneliness spoke to mine, and provided one moment of warm acknowledgement of real feeling in a ward of starched dummies.

Then one day, at our group therapy meeting, a new doctor was introduced to us. He looked very young and eager, dressed in what looked like a milkman's jacket. He was smiling and asked what we thought of psychiatrists. This was an entrée I had been waiting for for two months now. Without hesitation I looked at him and said: 'I think all psychiatrists should be strung from the ceiling.'

This led to the beginning of a lifelong relationship. He saw me almost daily for one hour's therapy or consultation. He seemed to recognize quite quickly in talking to me, and to my parents, that I had been wrongly diagnosed. He said I was eccentric, but otherwise normal. He pleaded my case, and took me off the medication. I was three months in that hospital and at last, thanks to him, I was released, although other doctors said: 'Look, you can tell she's mad from the way she laughs.'

We were married six months later, and we had a daughter nine months after that, who is now 29, a Buddhist and a dancer. And three years ago he died. It is said that his heart burst. He died suddenly, alone by the shore, looking into the sea, on the Island of Iona, where St Molaise, in whose cave I write this account, had trained for the priesthood.

I write this account, in part, in tribute to the memory of Graham Davies. His intelligence and courage in recognizing and affirming my eccentricity and sanity, and opposing the treatment in the face of vested medical establishment values and diagnosis, at the outset of his psychiatric training, was exceptional. He read natural sciences at King's College Cambridge, and studied medicine at University College Hospital. He trained subsequently at the Maudsley and Tavistock and under Gerda Boyeson. He was widely read in the arts and literature, and was familiar with the works of many philosophers and with the ideas and works of mystics. He was a loving husband and a loving father. His educational background in conventional and esoteric philosophy made it possible for him to distinguish between psychosis and other altered states of consciousness. I believe the concept that first made him recognize the truth of my spiritual as opposed to psychotic experiences was my description of the experience of white light, which he later experienced himself.

For those who have a real interest in consciousness (and that should include all healers involved in psychiatric care), it is imperative to study the works, accounts and descriptions of psychics, mystics, yogis, holy men, saints, mediums and spiritual healers, in order to understand their language and vocabulary as much as their experience. The language and universal vocabulary of altered states of consciousness can give one an indication of when psychosis is not the primary experiential status of a patient.

There is a level of self-consistency, self-insight and archetypal reference in the language of mysticism, certain key features of experience that characterize a spiritual awareness and transcendental state.

In schizophrenia, during a psychotic breakdown, thinking and perceptual processes are altered by being confused and fragmented, leading to an inability of the sufferer to carry out normal procedures – even eating and sleeping and washing. Paranoid delusions can take the place of objective reality. In order to understand the reality spoken of in mysticism, one has to stretch one's own understanding of objective reality – to undergo a willing suspension of disbelief. It takes humility to accept that much objective reality may in fact be hidden from many people, by dulled or conditioned perceptual processes.

My husband's life ended at the pinnacle of his career as a successful consultant psychotherapist and psychoanalyst, with many of his colleagues and patients testifying to his unique blend of Eastern and Western methods of probing states of consciousness and helping people attain synthesis. He had himself experienced mystical and altered states of consciousness during his lifelong training and practice.

I owe him my life, as I believe I was in mortal danger from the treatment I received before his advent. Had he not removed the medication, I may have sustained lasting liver and kidney damage, and had he not organized my speedy discharge, I might have become long-term institutionalized like Freddie. He gave me back my self-respect.

I went back to visit Freddie. He did not want to leave. He was happy tramping the grounds and long Victorian corridors, gazing at the water tower, and sometimes sleeping out all night in the fields, knowing that a warm bed and corrective treatment awaited him next day. He did not have to bother about socks or clocks. He did not have to see the woman who called herself his mother. (Needless to say, she was white.) He could live in his universe as God, and not have to face the cruelty and terror of the outside world.

Were it not for my rescue by my psychiatrist in shining amour, I would have been content to join Freddie there forever. It would have been a very long haul to rehabilitate me against my will.

My knight in shining armour has come home to Avalon, or to where it is reputed to be, near the grail of the healing Spring on Holy Island, next to the Cave of St Molaise, contemporary of St Columba of Iona, opposite the house where I was conceived by Kathleen and Cyril, fifty years ago.

And as I write and watch the rainbow stretching from the place of my conception to the healing spring, I affirm that I would like this to be a tribute and memorial to him.

Chapter 7
A Most Precious Thread

SIMON CHAMP

Editorial

Many people have tried, especially over the past fifty years, to draw comparisons between mental and physical illness; such comparisons almost normalize the experience of madness. We say almost, for Simon Champ's experience illustrates clearly how such comparisons can appear simplistic. However it is defined, most forms of mental illness are quite unlike physical illness. Whereas people have illnesses such as cancer or arthritis, Simon points out that a mental illness, especially in its more extreme form, appears to take over the whole person so that the person is the illness. If it does not actually do this, others are often keen to suggest that such a takeover has taken place. The fracture in the faith we normally have in our perceptions and thinking might incline us, after a severe psychotic episode, to accept such a view.

In A Most Precious Thread *Simon dismantles some of the standard thinking about schizophrenia, and attempts to rebuild a more realistic picture of this most human of conditions. Simon attempts to set his experience in context, examining what actually happens to a person when he/she is in schizophrenia, considering in what way such experiences are like, or unlike, the experiences known to the rest of us. Simon Champ reminds us that people who are defined, somewhat arbitrarily, as 'schizophrenics' are, more accurately, people who have highly specific and ultimately transient experiences of something that is defined, in this culture, as psychosis. Simon is reluctant to assign himself a passive, or suffering, role in relation to such experiences. The experience of psychosis, like the experience of everything else, is an active form of being. Experiencing psychosis is, in a sense, simply one of the things Simon Champ does. More importantly, he also has reflected, at length, on what those active experiences might mean for his relationship with himself, with his work and with his community.*

It is ironic, perhaps, that much of the discovery that Simon has made about his own human condition involves a deeper appreciation of its innate mystery. At a time when neuroscience is so anxious to close the book on schizophrenia, almost explaining it away with reference to various neurochemical hypotheses, it is refreshing to read about Simon's uncertainty in the face of this mysterious phenomenon. The awe that Simon experiences in the face of schizophrenia has clearly inspired him to look further. Here, he tries to clarify why, after many years of distress and life challenge, he still feels that his life has been enriched by the experience of psychosis. In doing so he clarifies for the reader, as well as himself, what exactly is the nature of the most precious thread that has sustained him down all those dark days.

★   ★   ★   ★   ★

A Most Precious Thread

I would like to achieve three things in writing this chapter. First, to reinforce to mental health professionals that a person experiencing schizophrenia can actively participate in his/her own recovery if encouraged and supported. It is only by engaging this participation that real recovery is accomplished. That is, real recovery is done *with* the person rather than *to* them.

Second, I hope that in trying to give form to these reflections about my own recovery, I will encourage nurses to help others who experience a mental illness to set down their own experiences of their process of recovery. I have often seen that there are still marked differences between what the mental health professional thinks is helping recovery and what that consumer knows works for him/her in recovery. Articulating the experience through such writing might not only resolve such differences, but can itself help recovery.

Finally, I write this because I have become increasingly concerned that, with the dominance of biochemical and physiological explanations of the schizophrenias, indeed of most mental illness, there is an increasing assumption that all you need to do for a person is to find the appropriate medication. My own journey with a whole range of different medications has taught me that medication is only one tool in recovery, that no one really recovers by medication alone. Real recovery requires counselling or therapy in addition to medication.

In Eastern religion there is a metaphor that says that one cannot step into the same river twice. Just as there is, in a sense, a new river, changing from moment to moment, so the flow of perceptions, thoughts and quality of being that is the experience of schizophrenia is in constant flux, evolving and never quite the same. There may be patterns to my delusions and remissions, common forms, but each time I am psychotic the delusions change, perhaps informed by the real events of my life. For me, schizophrenia is continually affecting me in new ways, changing in its intensity and forms. At times, it has seemed to have currents and seasons, but I have learned it has no rules. I have learned that there is no one strategy for minimizing the impact of the illness. Rather, the interventions need to be different at different times and sometimes used in conjunction with one another.

To live with this ever-changing experience of schizophrenia over 23 years has changed my relationship with myself many times and in many ways. I want to describe a few of these changes that have helped me deal with my schizophrenia. I want to reveal a little of the ongoing communication with myself that is a large part of my process of recovery.

For me, schizophrenia severely ruptured the relationship that I had enjoyed with myself prior to the illness. My sense of being in the world, my thought processes and, indeed, the very way my senses perceived the world would go through involuntary changes. I was plunged, at times, into a confusing and frightening world ruled by my own paranoias and delusions.

With my first psychotic episodes came many questions that have stayed with me in one form or another through all these years. I think sometimes professionals underestimate the psychological dislocation caused by even a single psychotic episode.

If your mind has played tricks, making you believe delusional thoughts, hearing or seeing things that are not real, then the first time you go into remission there can be a profound crisis. Prior to developing schizophrenia, the workings of my mind had been unquestioned. Suddenly I was being told by a psychiatrist that I could not always trust my own thoughts and senses. I felt that my own mind had betrayed me. How could I ever trust it? Self had become a traitor and was working against my own good.

If the realities I had lived in for some months were unreal, how could I believe that the reality I was currently experiencing was not another delusion? In the doubts and confusions of that period of adjustment I was also profoundly troubled by the implication that somewhere there must be states of mind that were 'normal'. If I had been 'insane', where was 'sanity'? As I looked out on the world after my delusions, it looked a very strange place with its starving millions, threat of nuclear accident, ecological crisis and the surreality of consumerism and popular culture.

The medications had changed how my very being felt to myself. The medications I was taking dulled my thoughts and robbed me of familiar emotions and feelings I had always known. The post-psychotic world seemed colourless in comparison with the world I had known before becoming ill. Trying to decide what was normal or sane was like negotiating a foreign city without a map. I felt like a stranger to myself.

Of course, over the years I have come to realize there is no 'normal' state. Rather, there are cultural conditionings and consensus views on what constitutes reality. Instead of these, I have sought states of mental wellbeing and ways of being in life that are meaningful for me. But in the confusion after my first episodes I searched for measures of sanity that were the opposite of the states of illness I had known. That search for some measure of 'normalcy' was doubly confusing as each health worker I encountered would tend to see the indicators of my progress differently. I had yet to learn for myself just how arbitrary are the standards by which people who do not experience a mental illness measure their own sanity, just how many value judgements were inherent in the way professionals treated me and the way they measured a consumer's quality of life.

The nurses I most valued at that time were those who, rather than impose their reality on me, helped me to explore where reality and wellbeing might exist for me.

Beyond the crisis of deciding which reality I would inhabit and wondering where sanity lay for me, the other profound challenge to my relationship with myself in my early remissions came from the lack of help to integrate the material that had manifested in my psychotic states. To go into remission after a psychotic episode is to gradually realize what I have thought, believed and done while I have been ill. Gradually, my memories of events would return and I was faced with seemingly bizarre, embarrassing and frightening thoughts and actions from my previous episode. The first few times I experienced psychotic episodes, I had a hard time coming to terms with what had passed through my mind or how I had acted. It was like recalling a nightmare, except that I had lived it out, manifesting it in the world. My thoughts and actions seemed so out of keeping with my character as I had known it that it was very hard to accept that I had actually experienced them. It seemed like another person or another life and, in retrospect, I can understand how people believe the 'split personality' myths or believe in possession to explain schizophrenia.

Gradually, and with much pain, I had to realize that these thoughts and actions were my own, even if they arose out of unknown places inside me.

I have learned over the years that it is only by owning and embracing this strange world within, from which the psychosis arises, that I have any chance of controlling its manifestations or preventing it from overwhelming me.

If a person has a powerful dream, particularly if it is a frightening dream, he/she tends to share it at breakfast with family, lover or friends. It is an acceptable practice that sometimes provides psychological insights and diminishes some of the fear the dream holds for the dreamer. However, symptoms of a mental illness frighten our colleagues and family, so the contents of delusion are still rarely shared or explored. The domination of biochemical theories of illnesses like schizophrenia has further stifled discussions about the often frightening contents of psychotic episodes. We are so often encouraged to repress the fears we feel from our symptoms or have the whole experience lost to the mental fog of higher doses of medication. I found that I needed to talk about the contents of delusions to dissipate the fear they held for me. The best staff allowed me to go over my psychotic experiences, gradually diffusing the power they held over me, and they helped me to integrate the delusions as best I could, into some sense of being whole and earthed again. I desperately needed to understand what psychosis was and extract some kind of meaning from the experience. I could only do that by telling it over many times.

If the onset and early years of living with schizophrenia radically changed my relationship with myself, that relationship was further changed by the treatments I received. When I was psychotic, I often perceived hospitalization and medication as a threat. Sometimes, as in one delusion when I believed that the hospital I was being held in was a concentration camp, where I was going to be gassed, I was terribly traumatized by the very interventions and professionals that were supposed to be helping me. Even when I went into remission, I often felt that my treatment was a punishment for being different.

The experience of hospitalization gave me lasting negative messages that took me years to really work through. Those messages were that I was unacceptable to society, that I was bad and that I had little power of my own. Those feelings for me are forever symbolized by the euphemistically called 'Time Out' rooms (solitary confinement), when I was least able to bear the terrible fears I was experiencing because of paranoia. I was locked away with those fears, away from other human beings who might have reassured or genuinely cared for me. It taught me that society wanted to lock away and isolate what it was most afraid of: extreme states of mental anguish. I think that this act alone, putting me in solitary confinement, confirmed my sense that I was an outsider to society. It left me bitter and deeply alienated, as did the rest of my first hospitalization. Being locked away seemed to enhance the feelings of guilt and shame I felt for having a mental illness.

During those first years of living with a diagnosis, I had a great struggle with my self-image, constantly putting myself down and having those feelings reinforced by the stigma in society. I even believed at times that my schizophrenia was a punishment from God for sins I could not remember. This was an idea reinforced by some Christians who told me that schizophrenia was, indeed, a punishment for sin. Other Christians went further, telling me that it was a form of possession.

Such experiences were certainly a low point in my life, but even at such times, somehow, I managed to keep a journal, a record of my days. Nowadays, as a national speaker on mental health issues, I carefully consider words I use and try to encourage politically correct, first-person language when talking about consumer experiences. So it is with much sadness for my younger self that I read, in the pages of those early diaries, my constant descriptions of myself as being 'a schizophrenic'. Now if I have to consider my illness as relevant to who I am, I would say 'I am a person who experiences psychosis', never simply labelling myself 'schizophrenic'. Beyond my ideological sensitivities, what saddens me, looking back to when I called myself 'a schizophrenic', is that in those early stages of adjusting to schizophrenia, my image of myself was dominated by the fact that I experienced the illness. For some time, my illness was central to my identity. I felt the illness would determine my life and most of my energies were consumed in a daily struggle with positive and negative symptoms of the illness. Sadly, I was my illness and, disempowered, I allowed myself to be described as 'a schizophrenic'.

So often I recall the period when, finally, that changed. It was the beginning of a long change in how I have come to understand my relationship with the illness schizophrenia. At a certain point I was so depressed with the prognosis for a schizophrenic illness and the literature I was reading about schizophrenia, that I began to think I would live my life as an experiment. I would try not to absorb the negative messages that I was reading about people who lived with schizophrenia, and would try, instead, to find out for myself what this diagnosis would mean for me in my own life. It was the beginning of a mental turn-about, trying to re-establish my life and find a more accurate sense of self.

For some time this change actually took the form of seeing people who experienced schizophrenia as being special: specially sensitized individuals, who could experience dimensions to the spectrum of human consciousness and spirituality that others, not affected, were not privileged to. At this time I wore the label 'schizophrenic' with pride and as a mark of distinction. I began something of a one-man crusade to redefine the term and give it dignity. During this period I celebrated the culture and history of people who had experienced schizophrenia and generally had a much more positive image of myself. However, my image of myself was still dominated by the fact that I had schizophrenia. In reality, I was having episodes of my illness every three to six months. Often I would proudly introduce myself: 'Hi, I'm Simon and I'm schizophrenic', offering a challenge to people I met to come to terms with the illness while I was busy redefining the illness and myself in the process.

Gradually, I came to see that it was damaging to refer to myself as 'a schizophrenic', both politically and for my own view of myself. Extended periods of remission, study at an art school and being involved in raising awareness about schizophrenia were giving me a much fuller life, and I had a greater sense of control over my symptoms. I was recovering my personhood and saw the illness as influencing, rather than defining me.

At this stage I began to see that, while I might not be able always to control my illness, I could control my attitude to it. I began to see strong links between quality of life and the attitude one had to illness. I became increasingly concerned by the language and attitudes expressed by many members of the Schizophrenia Fellowship of New South Wales, an organization I had helped start. The constant reference to people who experience schizophrenia as 'sufferers' and 'victims' of illness seemed offensive to me. While I was the first to admit that schizophrenia had dominated my life for many years and that it could, indeed, be a terrible disease, I also knew that I had only really made progress in my own recovery when I stopped seeing myself as a 'victim' and relinquished more passive roles in my treatment. 'Sufferer' was the language of victims and lacked dignity. Illness was becoming one aspect of a whole me, not the centre of me. By changing the focus of the illness in my life, I think my management of the illness was further strengthened. I was indeed a person who happened to experience psychotic episodes, but I refused to be described as a 'sufferer'.

Even for those of us facing great psychiatric disabilities, our souls can flower with hope. Hope is an essential ingredient for recovery. When I began experiencing schizophrenia, it was a great struggle to revive a sense of hope in my life. I felt spiritually abandoned by any notion of a God I may have had. For long periods, life seemed hopeless and my despair was exacerbated by my constant struggle with symptoms.

So many of the images of schizophrenia in literature, films and popular media gave me little hope. Often, when I met aged people who had experienced schizophrenia, their lives seemed depressing, lacking fulfilment. They hardly offered me inspiration. It was only later that I realized that, rather than seeing the long-term effects of illness, more often I was witnessing the effect of attitudes towards that illness. In their impoverished lifestyles and lives I was seeing not what medics explain as a kind of burn-out from schizophrenia, but the degradation of the spirit by poverty, neglect, stigma, over-medication, institutionalization and lack of opportunity. At first I did not understand that, and the memories of older patients I had seen in hospital and met in boarding houses depressed and frightened me. If that was my future, I did not want to live. At times I was in a dilemma because I did not want to live but was still afraid of death. It seemed at times that Earth had become my purgatory.

Hope has come in many forms, some surprising, some hard won over the years. In its absence I tried to manufacture it. Depression has always come as a result of psychosis, both as a 'physical' post-psychotic phenomenon, and as depression with origin in the disappointment and grief I experienced because of symptoms and stigma. Depressions could last months and I would desperately try to revive hope in those times. Gradually, through the years, I have learned some basic techniques to revive hope, using it as a resource in my life, a kind of account of the spirit.

The inner dialogues with self that have defined who I am are also influenced by my relationships in the outside world. While relationships with mental health professionals have sometimes helped this inner evolution, another influence has increased in significance for me over the years. My contact with other people who have experienced a mental illness, at first informally and later through the consumer movement, has profoundly influenced my relationship with myself,

When I was first experiencing schizophrenia, I would often feel alone and different. Meeting others who experienced schizophrenia taught me that, though I was part of a minority, I was still having symptoms and difficulties that were shared. It could give me hope to see others manage symptoms that still gave me difficulty. It was a relief to be able to share aspects of life and feelings that others knew from first-hand experience. It really helped to have my own feelings validated. The friendships with other consumers helped me to become more self-accepting and also gave me valuable insights and encouragement for the process of recovery I was engaged in.

Much has changed in mental health over last fifteen years – especially how consumers see themselves in relation to services. It is being said that 'the personal is political' and, for me, meeting other consumers ignited a passionate indignation at the societal injustice faced by people who have experienced a mental illness. That personal indignation has led to something of a career for me as an adviser and activist on mental health.

It was in the company of consumers that I really began to understand how stigma, poverty and a lack of rights, services and opportunity constrained my concept of self. While politically I became involved in moves towards empowerment of consumers, at a personal level I was trying to overcome the limited notions of self I had myself absorbed from society. Politically, consumers were stepping out of the shadows of shame and injustice, but I was surprised at how many places inside me were still darkened by my internalization of society's treatment and attitudes to people who had experienced a mental illness. They say of some depression that it can be anger turned inward. I also discovered during these times that, by expressing anger, hope is freed. As I worked through the anger I felt at the treatment I had received, I felt a renewed sense of hope for my own life.

Schizophrenia has changed my relationship with myself in some ways that are specific to people who experience mental illness. But sometimes, in dealing with schizophrenia, I have faced challenges to concepts of self that are experienced by other groups in our society. Two areas of my life that went through a redefinition because of my experience of schizophrenia, and which have relevance beyond the mental health field, were my identity in relation to work and my concept of my own masculinity.

In the early years of living with schizophrenia, I experienced major disruptions to my life and I was unable to do any regular form of work. Like many people who experience long periods of unemployment, my sense of self plummeted until eventually I began to redefine myself in relation to work. So often in our society we are viewed and fall into the trap of seeing ourselves through what we do for a living rather than who we are as a person. I had become not only a person who experienced mental illness, but also a recipient of welfare, unable to work. My sense of worth and value to society declined.

Some time later, I began to feel that I could contribute to life in other ways. Meaning and worth need not be generated solely by traditional forms of work, but could be extracted from the many other types of relationship and activity I could develop through the full part I might play in my community.

Nowadays, I enjoy work whenever I can and have found much fulfilment in finding ways to employ my talents. But having a disability has
changed the way I view myself as a worker in society and redefined the role
and value I attribute to work in my life. I am certainly not alone in this
transition, for in our economic climate there are many other people who do
not experience mental illness, who are also forced to redefine their
relationship to work.

One area I believe would benefit from more research is the link
between gender and the experience of schizophrenia: how the symptoms
and forms of schizophrenia might vary between men and women, and the
implications of such variance for treatment; the subtleties of differences in
the effects and side-effects of medications as experienced by men and
women.

The experience of schizophrenia has challenged me to redefine my
own concepts of masculinity. Upwellings of subconscious material in
psychosis, finding myself breaking down and losing control of emotions,
has expanded my notions of masculinity. I discovered that real men do
indeed cry and experience a whole range of emotions that need to be
expressed to maintain true mental health, especially if one has the
additional stress of a schizophrenic illness.

Many men who experience mental illness feel emasculated in some
way in their own eyes and those of their peers. I believe that this sense of
emasculation because of mental illness can be a factor, not usually considered, contributing to many young male suicides.

For some like myself, schizophrenia has actually been an opening,
even if painful one, into a wider conception of masculinity. I found some
support for this evolving conception in the writings of the men's
movement and men's groups, where there is a growing recognition that
traditional masculinities may actually exacerbate health problems,
including mental health problems for men.

Here I have touched on only some of the changing concepts of self I
have experienced through the many years I have been in recovery. Some
concepts have evolved, some are ongoing and some have fallen away. In
coming to terms with schizophrenia and recovering a healthier concept of
self, I have certainly been engaged in a deep communication with myself. It
is a communication that has given me the most precious thread, a thread
that has linked my evolving sense of self, a thread of self-reclamation, a
thread of movement toward a whole and integrated sense of self, away
from the early fragmentation and confusion I felt as I first experienced
schizophrenia.

Not everyone who experiences schizophrenia will question the concept of who they really are in the same ways that I have. Nevertheless, I believe most will be profoundly challenged to redefine concepts of self because of the illness.

I have come to see that you do not simply patch up the self you were before developing schizophrenia, but that you have to actually re-create a concept of who you are that integrates the experience of schizophrenia. Real recovery is far from a simple matter of accepting diagnosis and learning facts about the illness and medication. Instead, it is a deep searching and questioning, a journey through unfamiliar feelings, to embrace new concepts and a wider view of self. It is not an event but a process. For many, I believe it is a lifelong journey.

I am lucky that I have always had an interest in art and journal writing. Both have helped me pass through the stages of my recovery. In a daily diary, I was able to have a dialogue with self in which I have examined some of the pain, surprise and joys of the transformations I have been through. The diaries have always been with me, a 24-hour confidant, mirror of self and adviser. They were available in the loneliness and terror of paranoid nights and empty weekends when mental health workers were not available. I have gradually learned through keeping the diary that I have more wisdom and insight about schizophrenia than I ever initially believed possible, if only I manage to reconnect with the story of my own life and feelings contained in the diary.

The diary and my paintings externalize the inner communications that I am constantly engaged in, which integrate the experience of schizophrenia into my life and help control its symptoms. They are vehicles for working through the complex emotions that have arisen during stages of my recovery: feelings of despair and helplessness, when I thought life was not worth living because I did not understand schizophrenia; feelings of anger and being cheated by life because I had an illness that caused such disruption; feelings of failure because I had relapsed again. These and many other feelings I would gradually understand, integrate and turn around through my art and writing.

Some of this was done privately, on my own, but some of the professionals who have supported me in my journey have seen the value of these creative endeavours in my overall treatment.

I think the best professionals involved in my care have walked alongside me, opening themselves to the mystery that is schizophrenia. They have gained my trust, sharing and supporting my inner search for meaning and understanding of self in relation to illness. We have certainly learned about medication, but we have also learned to predict stressors and avert relapse, seeing my well-being as a result of many influences on my life. They have helped me try to integrate the strange upwellings of psychotic material and to deal with the fear and unease caused by relapse. They have not always been certain but, rather, experimenters like myself, carefully watching what was happening at a specific time with my own particular form of schizophrenia, before choosing an intervention.

While putting together thoughts for this chapter, my diary has been beside me, observer and commentator. To draw to a close, I would like to share two entries from my diaries, written while preparing this chapter. The first reflects some of the emotions and memories that were stirred up for me, and a flashback from some 15 years ago.

Wednesday 2 July 1997

Today, more notes for the chapter as I reflect on what is the nature of my relationship to myself, that precious thread that has evolved after 23 years of living with this illness that has been diagnosed as paranoid schizophrenia. There are psychological theories about how the oppressed begin to identify with the oppressor. At the early stages of my illness, the nurses were the oppressors of my mind, agents of social control in my paranoid world-view, enforcers of mediocrity and the status quo. I called the nurses 'soul fuckers', for the medication seemed to eat at my very soul. They were the ones that administered the injections, the 'mind death'.

As I write the chapter I borrow forms learned from the language of psychology and psychiatry that I've come to know too well. I don't want to make myself into my own 'case study'. It's a form of searching for acceptance, writing like that; yes, and identification with the oppressor. How well I have learned compliance.

How can I honestly talk of the inner self, 20 years ago paranoid and psychotic with an inner language that had meanings all of its own? How inadequate words seem to express the anger, frustration and fear of those times when my mind clawed its way free of psychotic episodes; the terror when you're alive but pinch yourself to see if you are real and then find you don't exist.

How strange notes in an old hospital file seem: Nurses observing my inner hell. The notes seem irrelevant. It's another person, not me. How can one human know the reality of another? ...when paranoia and fear break communication with the observer, the recorder in his nurses' station, break communication even from myself. Lost from myself.

The second entry from my diary celebrates my new-found well-being and shows that, after 23 years, though I have gained more control over schizophrenic symptoms, the illness is more of a mystery to me now than it ever was.

Sunday 12 July 1997

Why am I so blocked, unable to write this chapter? Is it because of late I am so well, better than I've ever been before, that I just want to enjoy well-being and forget the traumas of the past; that I want to get on with my life, free of symptoms, with even the negative symptoms improved; so well I can stand on new ground that gives a clearer view than I've ever had of my life? From here I can see for the first time clearly the difficult path I've followed and glimpse new horizons ahead. But in looking back now from this vantage point of mental well-being, I mourn the years lost to this illness. I wonder what could have been. I've never known this kind of freedom from schizophrenia, the irony that I've adapted to having such an illness. This new well-being demands adjustment too. I know how to live with schizophrenia – I don't yet know how to live with this kind of well-being. Do I dare to hope and plan in new ways? Sometimes, with the schizophrenia, I'm so used to an ambience of paranoia in my days that I don't notice it until it becomes an absence. The absence of something that was the residual effect of schizophrenia is a feeling of ease, a piece of mind that I've never known before. In some way it feels as if I've come home to myself, a self changed, a self I last felt at 17, and yet now I'm 40. All those years of experiences separate me from the teenager I was, but somewhere inside I'm complete again, as I used to be then. In between, despite having schizophrenia, I've lived a full life. So what was missing? What has returned? What is that quality of being, so hard to define, that is an essential part of what I'm trying to understand for this chapter, a kind of being-in-the-world, -in-reality?

Somewhere there's a thread, a precious thread that runs and connects through some twenty years, that has led me home to myself.

Recently, talking to my friend Helen, who also started feeling so much better on the same medication I switched to six months ago, she said of the medication 'it gives you back your mind'. The drug company would love that as a testimony, I'm sure.

Now that's part of the conflict as I write, that I am unsure how to attribute my new-found well-being. I believe the new medication has helped, as has all the 'work' I do on myself and, perhaps, as has been suggested by some researchers, the fact that the illness moderates with age or you better learn how to manage the symptoms. But in what measure has each of these factors contributed to this dramatic improvement I'm experiencing?

And what is the thread through the years?

In conclusion, perhaps the newer medications for schizophrenia will make for a smoother journey of reintegration for younger people now being diagnosed with a schizophrenic illness. Perhaps their journeys will be very different from mine, a little easier. I hope so.

Ultimately, even a paranoid delusion is a miraculous thing, testimony to the infinite wonder that is the human mind. Learning to integrate such bizarre phenomena into my life and still find meaning has enriched my life, for all its hardships.

Quite often, I have had other people who experience schizophrenia come up to me, after I have given a talk about the illness, and, as if confessing, say in a secretive tone that they believe their schizophrenia is a gift.

Only on my good days do I think my schizophrenia is a gift. More often, it is an awe-inspiring mystery that begs many questions. I hope that some of you reading this will find ways to answer those questions.[5]

---

[5] This chapter previously appeared in the Australia and New Zealand Journal of Mental Health Nursing 1998 (7) 54–59. Reproduced with permission.

Chapter 8
Hope, Humanity and Voice in Recovery from Mental Illness

DAN FISHER

Editorial

Not too many research scientists have come out of the closet of madness, while even fewer psychiatrists have emerged from the same closet. In these circumstances, Dan's story is a fascinating one. Dan believes that his honesty about his experience of madness is the key to his own recovery.

Dan's story is not, however, just about 'coming out' and encouraging like-minded people to join him. His journey into and beyond madness is characterized by his discovery of him-self in the process, and in his steadfast refusal to look outside of that self – the 'me' that becomes 'I' – for explanations, far less blame, for the human details of his breakdown. In that sense, Dan Fisher is one of that growing band of individuals who are taking back the personal power that the various processes of madness and treatment appeared to have taken from them. Parents, families and culture are easy targets for those seeking something to blame for their misfortune. Indeed, much psychotherapeutic practice has focused on locating and rooting out such factors, as part of the recovery process. Dan suggests the value in turning our backs on this blame-culture, advocating a kind of compassion that may, ultimately, bring true healing.

The way that Dan has reclaimed his own territory finds an echo in many others who, once defined as patients, have redefined themselves as users, consumers and prosumers. All such titles may represent a march back to the adoption of personhood that seems to lie at the heart of Dan's thesis. The 'person robbery' apparently effected by madness is revealed in Dan's story to be largely illusory but, nonetheless, a significant factor in the deprivation many 'patients' feel in respect of self-determination and responsibility. Dan shows how person-hood can never be stolen, as long as the spirit remains. That human spirit lies waiting for the opportunity to reveal itself, so that the person may ultimately reveal him- or herself.

For Dan, the processes of madness involve a frustrating (or maddening) provocation of the person's true identity, but also an opportunity for it to develop. The robbery of selfhood is thus perhaps a paradoxical challenge to develop true personhood. In that curious sense, Dan Fisher's story recalls Epictetus' dictum that 'difficult circumstances do not so much ennoble, as reveal a person'. As a psychiatrist, his story also serves as another experiential echo of Frankl's thoughts when he was brought to the edges of his own physical self by his Nazi medical torturers: 'No matter what they do to me, they can never touch me.'

Dan reminds us of the need to remember that, whatever may befall a person, within that person resides a voice of human reason that is waiting to make contact. Perhaps the first contact needs to be with a source of help, but ultimately its aim is to make contact with the 'me' that is the social-self. Once the 'I' of the spirit is united with the 'me' of the self, then an opportunity for human wholeness can declare itself.

★   ★   ★   ★   ★

I see a spirit in the eyes and hearts of others who have recovered from mental illness. It is a force that drove us to recover. It connects us with the life we all are part of. It is an inspiration. We emerge from the shadows with a message for all humanity. The time has come to unite in the greatest struggle we as a people have ever encountered. It is a struggle to see if we can put aside our prejudices and if we can continue our interrupted evolution towards being human, whole, and connected with each other and with the world. Our journeys are uniquely our own. There are, however, certain themes, principles and values that continually emerge. The three I will emphasize here are hope, humanity and voice.

I no longer search for the sickness in myself or in those I grew up with as an explanation for my woes. Instead I search for the strengths in myself and those close to me which propel me through my version of the suffering we all share but seldom face. I, psychiatry and our society need to shift away from our current perspective, featuring negative feedback and a pathological emphasis on *external locus of control*; we should shift toward a person-driven, democratic, *internal locus of control perspective.*

I was the third child in a 'professional' family of four children in Baltimore. Born 50 years ago, during a popular war, I grew up in a time of plenty. There was a predictability and security in the place where my mother still lives, which nourished optimism. There was the bomb in the background and we talked about it. But we had hopes that world peace could be achieved through disarmament. I was a Unitarian. I could play an active role in the shaping of that world. I have always felt in darkest times that there is a *me* inside that I can draw upon.

My mother was always asking questions of herself and of me, which kept me searching for deeper truths. My father was a doctor, who told me stories of his childhood and had a caring approach to his patients when I went on rounds with him at the hospital (not fully understanding what I saw). I was a peacemaker in my family. I looked for ways to help people get along. When I experienced several traumas in my early teens (several reversals in love and my father developing a progressive disease), I turned to silence as a way to gain control and to fix these problems.

I became a biochemist. I thought I could understand why people became unhappy by a study of brain chemistry. I did not realize that it was my own unhappiness I needed to deal with first. I went to do research with a biochemist who headed the Lab of Neurochemistry at NIMH. He was convinced that you should be able to write a formula for every aspect of life.

Together we studied the enzymes regulating the production of the neurotransmitters dopamine, serotonin and norepinephrine. After five years of work, I had found at least 40 different variables, such as heat, oxygen, salt and iron, which profoundly affected the activity of those enzymes. I was able to make these discoveries by getting into the problem. In fact, at one point I got so far into the problem that I became convinced that I was the enzyme I was studying. I could literally see the chemicals attaching to the enzyme (me) and could see them transformed into new chemicals. Later I felt reduced further to a slow-moving electron. I felt fragmented and lost. I became very fearful and was ordered into the psychiatric ward of Bethesda Naval Hospital across the street from my lab at NIMH (as a member of the Public Health Service I did not require a hearing to be committed).

I did a lot of thinking as I looked through the screened windows to the red-brick buildings of NIMH across the street. I realized that all those chemicals in me needed some greater sense of direction. I felt 'like a rolling stone/a complete unknown/no direction home', as Bob Dylan described it. Without meaning or identity, the enzyme I worked with and all the other millions of enzymes in my body were subjected to the whims of hundreds of stimuli each day. This was the inner process determining my experience of madness. I realized that I could not individually control each reaction, as I had hoped. I needed to find a collective, artistic approach to becoming a person.

I joined an acting group, and I learned modern dance. I later gained great support from a square-dancing group. These activities provided a unique opportunity for me to meet new people, join a community and express myself creatively. The sense of expression and connection I felt with the group opened my eyes.

I found a young, eclectic therapist and I made one request of him, 'Could you be a *real person* in your work with me?' He respected my request by sharing stories of his own sufferings as a child. He stated repeatedly that I had the capacity to heal myself and that he merely provided a setting for me to do that work.

All these developments soon collided with my life in the laboratory. I experienced a clash between my discovery that I needed human contact – at a deep level – to continue my recovery, and the impersonal laboratory work. I tried to resolve this conflict by returning to school to become a psychiatrist.

I next found a group therapist who taught me a great deal about how to understand myself in relation to others. During this period I had a dream of gaining freedom from my fear of authority:

> In the dream I saw two Corporals held captive in a castle. Whenever they tried to leave, their captor, a Colonel, would show them a picture of a gargoyle which he said looked like the corporals' brains. The corporals were then forced to return to their scientific work. A Lieutenant arrived and studied why the Corporals were there. He discovered that they had been looking through a microscope too long and had developed blind spots. The damage had reversed, however. The three presented the new information to the Colonel who kept pulling out his pictures of gargoyles. The Corporals and Lieutenant brushed him aside and, together, they left the castle, to emerge in sunlight.

This dream reinforced hope and pointed to my need for friends to help me build a positive image of myself. I believe that this dream predicted my transition from a *coping* to a *healing* phase of my recovery. I was not yet ready, however, for the sunlight.

I became convinced that we were all machines and I was rehospitalized. As an extension of my mechanized view of life, I became convinced that my emotional problems were caused by permanent organic damage to my brain. I felt I was being returned to the castle of fear and placed under the Colonel's influence. I was ready to abandon all hope of recovery. My therapist, however, continued to believe in my capacity to heal. In that dark hour, as I despaired on an inpatient unit, my therapist said that he did not think that my problems were organic and he still felt that I could heal. He demonstrated his trust in my capacity to face my problems by releasing me before I was fully co-operating with the staff. He helped me keep hope alive till I could hope for myself again.

After I left hospital, I felt I could not continue in medical school. Yet I did not want to disappoint my parents. I asked them to come down and visit. I tearfully told them that I didn't feel that I could go on in school. They said I should do whatever would make me the happiest. That statement gave me a great feeling of freedom, and allowed me to make the decision I thought would be best for me. I talked to some friends and decided that I wanted to continue medical school after all. A few days later I asked myself if I really wanted to go on struggling and I said 'Yes, to life', because I felt I was now living my own life, not someone else's. This emergence of hope for me is similar to Pat Deegan's (1993) description of the moment of grace in her recovery.

For many parents who have children with severe emotional problems, the concept that their emotional turmoil and vulnerability result from a 'mental illness', and that illness is caused by a chemical imbalance, is a source of reassurance. In circumstances where many parents have been unjustly accused of being responsible for their child's suffering, the 'no-guilt, chemical model' is a welcome relief from the model sometimes described in psychodynamic theories. For my part, I seek to find a common ground between the camps of consumers, family members and professionals where each group can understand the meaning of the other's views and agree not to impose theirs on the other.

I do not find the neurobiological theory of mental illness as helpful to my recovery because it deprives me of any sense of self-determination and responsibility. When I think that I am a group of chemical reactions, each with its own scheme and plan, I feel dehumanized and powerless. I feel that I am thinking, feeling and acting at the whim of those chemicals, not through any effort or responsibility of my own. A parent of an individual diagnosed as mentally ill captured this frustration when she told me, 'I am tired of hearing that what we do is the result of chemical imbalances. My son sits and says he cannot get up from his chair because of his chemical imbalance. He has no sense of responsibility for his life.' In addition, she was distressed that, as a consequence of that view, all her own accomplishments were merely the result of her chemicals being in balance, not due to her own efforts. This mechanical view also robs *me* of hope. If I feel there is nothing I can do or understand about my condition to help me to improve, I feel hopeless.

I do not find it helpful to say that mental illness is caused by a chemical imbalance. A number of consumers have come to me and said that they were told that their problems were due to a chemical imbalance and they should take medication for the rest of their lives. I suggest that they should try therapy, a consumer-run drop-in centre, a clubhouse or supported employment to carry out their recovery. They say all they need to do is take their medication. They do not see the point of these other activities, since their problem was described to them as chemical. Another problem with this mechanical view is that it removes people from their unique histories, relationships, classes and cultures. Yet these have been shown to be some of the most important variables both in aetiology of and recovery from mental illness.

E. Fuller Torrey, MD, now, paradoxically, a spokesperson for the biological model of mental illness, wrote an excellent book in 1980, *Schizophrenia and Civilization* which convincingly showed that cultural and social factors play a dominant role in the manifestations of and in recovery from extreme mental states diagnosed as schizophrenia. I will briefly summarize one of the articles he cited in his review:

> Dr Burton-Bradley, an Australian psychiatrist, spent 15 years in New Guinea, where he saw over a thousand cases of psychiatric disturbance in the indigenous people. He found that 'The person of limited (western) cultural contact, the so-called *bush* individual, very rarely presents with the symptoms of schizophrenia. This would suggest that the sociocultural influence of the town, with the confusing effect of alien values, may act as a precipitating factor in a predisposed person, and give rise to overt schizophrenia. This hypothesis is further supported by the fact that this condition often arises within the first few months of town life, and often readily resolves on return to the village. (1980, p. 81)

In summary, I would like briefly to state my view of the essential aspects of recovery: There is inside of me a self, a spirit, which is gradually becoming more aware of me and others. That self is becoming my guide. It encompasses all that I am. My self includes, but is greater than, my chemicals, my background and my traumas. It is the me I am seeking to become in my relationships, in that moment of creative uncertainty when I make contact with another. From that moment of harmony, when, together, we defy the odds and say 'yes', our lives will go on differently, regardless of how we live the following moment. We are all inventing our lives at each moment.

I hope... and a bridge appears to a future with other people.
I feel connected to humanity... and I find my voice.
I speak... and my voice breathes new life to sustain me and those I love.[6]

Reference

Deegan PE (1993) Recovering our sense of value after being labelled. Journal of Psychosocial Nursing 31: 7–11.
Torrey EF (1980) Schizophrenia and Civilization. New York: Jason Aronson.

---

[6] This copyright material is reprinted by special permission from the publisher of The Journal of the California Alliance for the Mentally Ill. It is part of a 28 article issue entitled Recovery available from The Journal/CAMI, 111 Howe Avenue, Suite 475, Sacramento, CA 95825.

Chapter 9
My Three Psychiatric Careers

RACHEL E. PERKINS

Editorial

We are all more alike than different, but, in the way we are different, we are unique. The idea that we are any one thing, whether we call it personality, identity or character, is illusory. But the business of living and relating helps us to develop the unique dimensions of ourselves, each of which might say something about who we are and what we are becoming.

Rachel Perkins is another author in this text who straddles the divide between being a provider and a recipient of mental health services. This dual status is extended further, in Rachel's case, by a third dimension, that of a campaigner, or social activist. Her appreciation of her multidimensional, or changing, nature may not be unusual, but her willingness to share her appreciation of her three careers with others is part of her uniqueness. We need more people, like Rachel, who can look at themselves from their many differing but related vantage points, seeing the connections, but also seeing the differences.

As with some of the other stories told in this book, Rachel challenges the myth of the 'suffering' of people with mental health problems, and the misconception that such human problems are necessarily all bad, or are not, in some way useful. She also addresses the often vexed issue of 'traditional' treatments – medication and ECT – versus some of the 'softer', psychological treatments available. As a psychologist, what she has to say about the relationship between 'medical' and 'psychological' interventions is particularly significant.

The usefulness of a senior mental health service 'provider' reflecting on the experience of being a mental health service 'recipient' can hardly be overstated. When those two careers flow into a third career as social activist, then the reader may begin to appreciate the potential dialogue between these separate, yet related, domains of experience for all people who deliver, receive or campaign about mental health services.

★ ★ ★ ★ ★

My Three Psychiatric Careers

I yelled at them when they came to see me. I yelled for some time. I really did not want to hear what my two best friends had to say. They told me they thought there was something wrong with me. The sort of something that meant I should see a psychiatrist. I was not pleased ... but after a while I began to see that they might have a point. Perhaps some of the problems I was having with work, with people, with meeting commitments, resulted not from my utter hopelessness and uselessness (as I had supposed) but from the fact that something was wrong. Perhaps if I saw a psychiatrist as they suggested, then there might be some light at the end of the tunnel. It took me some while to come to this conclusion, but when I did I found it somewhat liberating. For a while I could receive the absolution I needed for failing to do the things I usually did. My relationships with friends and family improved: I had not simply become lazy, unreliable and extremely irritable, now there was something 'wrong'. And anyway, why should I, who had been employed in mental health services all my working life, be so aggrieved that someone had suggested I might need such services myself?

Since 1980 I have had a career as a provider of mental health services, rising to the lofty heights of 'consultant clinical psychologist' in the rehabilitation field. In addition to my 'day job' I have a second 'career' as a campaigner and writer within the mental health field, especially in relation to services for women and lesbians, and those who are seriously disabled by their mental health problems. Over the years there had always been times when I had found work inexplicably and uncharacteristically hard – very, very hard; when I would burst into tears at the slightest provocation; when I would become irritable with everyone from friends and family to my colleagues and junior staff. I had been to GPs: one prescribed long walks which, needless to say, I did not take. But until 1992 I had not been accorded a label of madness.

The beginning of my third 'psychiatric career', as a recipient of mental health services, was quite different from the other two. It involved no positive choice on my part. You do not decide to become a psychiatric patient: apply for the position as you might for a job, or elect to join as you might a campaigning group. There are no guidelines about how to be a recipient of mental health services. No one tells you the rules as in a job description. Despite my long association with mental health services I found myself completely at sea, not really knowing what to do and feeling very alone. There were people around, but somehow I could not make contact with them as I usually did. An intangible barrier seemed to divide us.

From the accounts of others I thought I knew about the discrimination that the role of psychiatric patient attracts, although until I started to experience some of these things myself I did not know how desperate and hopeless I would feel. The relief brought by knowing 'something was wrong' was rapidly tempered by very real fear. What do I say to my friends? What do I tell them at work? What will happen to my (hitherto successful) career as a service provider? Or, at a micro level, there are the embarrassed encounters when I bump into former colleagues when I am in hospital or the psychiatrist's waiting room. There is, too, the way in which the look on the face of the chemist at the end of the street changes when I hand him my prescription for antidepressants and mood stabilizers ... and his refusal to sell me paracetamol. Other people had to collect the prescriptions for me for some time, and when first I dared to go myself I would only go to a large impersonal chain store where I would not, I thought, be recognized. For several months I shut myself away from all but my closest friends and relations. My sister and best friend looked after me – I could not manage alone and I was terrified of going into hospital. To make matters worse, my oldest and closest friend, who had been staying with me to support me, was killed in a cycling accident shortly after she left my flat. I could see little reason for staying alive myself.

I was off sick for almost six months, but gradually, with the love, help and support of my friends and family, and with the aid of drugs (the first in a long series of antidepressants and mood stabilizers that I have taken) I got back to work. Since then I have returned to this terrible pit on several occasions. Twice I have been admitted to hospital and twice I have chosen to have ECT because I could not bear to be in that place for long: with ECT I can get back to my life more quickly (I have written about this in more detail elsewhere – see Perkins, 1994). Throughout, the most important thing to me has been the support of my friends and relations. They make sure that someone visits me every day when I am in hospital; that someone is with me when I am at home; that they keep an eye on any treatment which is proposed – and ask all the questions that my sluggish thoughts cannot conjure.

I cannot separate the influence of my different associations with the mental health enterprise – my three psychiatric careers as provider, campaigner/writer and recipient of services – nor would I want to. My experiences in each are intimately interrelated and can be understood only in the context of all three. However, it was the third career as a recipient of services that was to change my relationship to the mental health services far more than I could ever have imagined.

On the Issue of Suffering

Life over the years since official confirmation of my madness has not been doom and gloom. In a review of one of my books (Webb, 1997) I was referred to as 'a sufferer': a description that I find singularly inappropriate. To describe oneself as 'a sufferer' implies that one's experiences are exclusively negative – that given a choice one would rather not have them.

It is true that I detest my depressions. I cannot make my thoughts work – it is like thinking through treacle. This is what bothers me most. I am used to thinking quickly, making decisions easily, working very hard, getting a kick out of driving my sports car. I enjoy the company of others and almost always have something to say! When my depression is at its worst I cannot make even the simplest choices about things such as what to wear. I cannot follow conversations, I cannot drive, I cannot work, I am totally unrewarding to be with. Once I spent over half an hour in a shop trying to decide which pack of lettuce to buy ... I failed and simply ran home feeling totally useless. Over the years I have found that just about the only thing I can do when I am in such a state is to knit: the pattern tells me exactly what to do, the work in front of me tells me what I have done. At these times I don't feel miserable or unhappy as in the colloquial use of the term 'depressed'. I know that I am useless and worthless, but I don't feel anything very much at all. The only reason for staying alive is that I will not be like this forever.

However, I would also contend that my manic depression is responsible for a great deal of the positive energy and creativity in my life. For a great deal of the time I am blessed with buckets of energy – more than most people. I love to work hard. My thoughts work like liquid crystal. I can see what things mean quickly and clearly. Ideas – generally good ideas – come to me with little or no effort when I need them. I know my surfeit of energy can be irritating to others, but my brain does all the things I want it to very efficiently and I am proud of it. I feel extremely engaged with, and part of, life. That I can do these things is not merely privately asserted but has been publicly recognized. Since gaining a diagnosis of manic depression I have been promoted to the position of clinical director (the only non-psychiatrist in my Trust to have such a role); been awarded a Churchill Fellowship; had a key role in developing a national Women and Mental Health Network; secured funding to instigate several mental health service developments; published over 50 papers; written two books and edited one. My co-author was most concerned when I started to take lithium. She said she was scared that we might stop having the wonderful conversations full of the energy and ideas that have fuelled our work together.

When I say things like this, it sounds like bragging. Sometimes I feel a need to brag. The first time I was billed to speak as a service user I felt an overwhelming desire to tell the audience about all my qualifications and achievements: 'Look, I'm not *just* a service user, I'm a clever professional as well'. Although I avoided this temptation, I do think that bragging is important on occasions. Everyone is always quick to point out the trials and tribulations of madness, the costs of madness, what madness *stops* people doing. Learned literature speaks of the distress and disability of madness, the burden of those who are mad on their kin in particular and on society in general. Underlying all talk of symptoms lies the assumption that they are bad things and must be eliminated. Yet this is a very partial picture. There is too little information on the contribution mad people make to our communities. I can tell of the awfulness and incapacity of depression, but this is only a fraction of my life and my madness. The benefits must also be counted. The different facets of my madness and moods are intimately interlinked, two sides of the same coin. I suspect that without one I cannot have the other. As Kay Jamison (1995) has so eloquently expressed:

> I have often asked myself whether, given the choice, I would choose to have manic depressive illness. ...Strangely enough I think I would choose to have it. It's complicated. Depression is awful beyond words or sounds or images.... So why would I want anything to do with this illness? Because I honestly believe that as a result of it I have felt more things, more deeply; had more experiences, more intensely; loved more, and been loved; laughed more often for having cried more often; appreciated more the springs, for all the winters; worn death 'as close as dungarees', appreciated it – and life – more; seen the finest and the most terrible in people, and slowly learned the values of caring, loyalty and seeing things through.

Those who are not mad prefer the idea that madness is exclusively a disabling and distressing thing. The thought that madness may have some positive features is possibly more threatening. That someone who is mad could actually be successful, not *despite* that madness but *because* of it, might actually mean that the stock responses of pity or condemnation are inappropriate. After all, if those labelled mad are as valuable as those labelled sane, what value in sanity? If there is such a thing as a gene increasing a person's risk of becoming mad, should we work out ways of ensuring that more people get it rather than trying to eliminate it, along with the energy and creativity which it brings?

A Fortunate Woman

'It's all right for you, you're different', 'You don't understand what it's like for everyone else', I have been told. Typically, such statements have come from people who wish to challenge my perspective on either the nature of my difficulties or appropriate remedies. They are particularly rife amongst those who disagree with my concerns about psychological and 'talking' therapies (Perkins, 1991; Kitzinger and Perkins, 1993). In any event, the position is flawed; one should start from the premiss that no one can know the experiences of another in the same way that they know it themselves and it is always arrogant for anyone, including professionals, to assume that they do. Therefore it is quite true that, in many ways, I am different (as is everyone else). However, I make no apologies for having been fortunate.

Most importantly I am blessed with wonderful friends and a family to whom I am close. Although I have lost some friends, most have been there for me in very real and material ways when I have not been able to cope, while always seeing me as an essentially competent and worthwhile person. This latter aspect is important. The quality of friendships and relationships does not lie solely in their ability to support at times of distress and difficulty. If this were the case, then such connections would simply nurture weakness and incompetence. Instead, relationships must also be able to celebrate and foster skills, strengths and competences. In my experience, most people who experience madness are strong and resourceful – they have to be to survive.

My experience of mental health services has been privileged. One of my best friends is a psychiatrist. She arranged for me to see a psychiatrist. A woman. A woman who had experienced similar mental health difficulties to my own. She was extraordinarily helpful and understanding. She seemed to know how I was feeling even when I could not find the words to tell her. Since she moved away I have another psychiatrist. She has always treated me rather as a colleague. Understood my need for information. Always given me chapter and verse on the research evidence for any recommendations she makes ... and left me to make the choices. On both occasions when I have been admitted to hospital I have had my own room.

Needless to say, everything has not been a bed of roses. I get angry, very angry, when I am treated as though I am stupid ('What is that?' – 'It's a drug that will make you feel better.'). But in general I have been more fortunate than many who have experienced problems such as mine. I work for the NHS. I am one of its own. A senior one of its own. My provider status changes my relationship with other professionals when I am using services. I am one of them. Here but for the grace of God go they. My status as a campaigner/writer means that I can and do recount my experiences as a recipient of services in talks, papers and books – a fact that might focus the mind of at least some of those who provide me with services. But my experiences do show that, where there is a will, good, largely respectful treatment is possible. Unfortunately it is this will that is so often sadly lacking.

The Nature of Madness

It is in the area of differing constructions of madness that I have probably experienced most dilemmas. It seems obvious to me that different explanatory models make sense to different people and that these different models, whether explicit or implicit, determine both the way in which people see and deal with their madness and the type of help they seek (Perkins and Repper, 1996). Different models of madness derive from different constructions of the world and events within it, but none is 'true' in any absolute sense. There is nothing 'truer' about assorted neurotransmitters than there is about intrapsychic processes, inner children or various deities. However, these different models do have different political and social implications and therefore debates between them are entirely appropriate.

My own constructions? Both my parents were natural scientists. When I was a child our house was often full of scientists, some from far-flung corners of the globe. A fascination with experiments – what, why and how things worked – embellished my childhood world. For me, science was delightful, elegant, sexy. It is not surprising, therefore, that I choose explanations for my madness in scientific terms. I am more comfortable with neurotransmitters than I can ever be with ids and egos, spiritualism and new-age mythology (Coward, 1989; Perkins, 1991; Kitzinger and Perkins, 1993).

But I was in a minority in a number of the domains that I inhabit.

My psychology colleagues were appalled that one of their number should opt for drugs and then ECT rather than the 'cognitive behaviour therapy' (or other psychological interventions) that our profession has invented. I have described my reasons for rejecting such approaches elsewhere (Perkins, 1991; Kitzinger and Perkins, 1993). Suffice here to say that I do not believe that, in general, my thoughts and belief systems are 'dysfunctional' and, where they are, changing my mind is the province of political discussion and debate, not therapy. The major problems that I experienced with my thoughts when depressed related not to their content but to their operation. It was not primarily that I thought about myself and the world in particularly negative terms, rather that I had difficulty in thinking about anything at all. When I spoke about my experiences at a 'Psychology of Women' conference, the large audience wore empathic expressions on their faces but refused to engage with what I was saying. When pushed, some said that I would have been better having the therapy which they asserted 'most people' want – a way of invalidating my viewpoint (by implication, you are not like 'most people'). I also heard several of these women psychologists ask of my friends 'Is Rachel *really* all right?' (If I was still 'mad' then my views could be discounted.)

Those with whom I campaigned on women's mental health issues often prefer to think in terms of psychotherapy, crystals, alternative therapies, spiritualism. Many were horrified when I decided to take drugs, and even more so when I decided to have ECT. While many espoused the importance of supporting other women in their decisions, it appears that these decisions too often have to be the 'right ones'. Far from supporting me in my decisions, I found some women at least as prescriptive as the traditional 'medical model' which they condemned. Several persisted in telling me of the error of my ways, and withdrew when I did not listen. Others, in a less extreme fashion, resumed contact with me only when I was 'better'. I lost some friends and allies, but I gained others and the quality of the relationships I had with those who remained with me was enhanced. To this day I have to struggle with the contradictions of being centrally involved in an organization whose newsletter (*Women and Mental Health Forum*) and membership frequently criticize as oppressive to women the treatments I have chosen.

It seems to me that there is a confusion between the prescriptive power of doctors and that which they prescribe. The power that doctors have to enforce treatment may be harmful, but this does not mean that all of the things that they prescribe are intrinsically bad: the real issues are about power and control, not drugs *per se*. Many feminists and other service users do opt to take drugs, but often avoid discussing this because of the accepted wisdom in such circles that 'drugs are a bad thing', 'drugs do not get to the root of the problem' (whatever that might be). By avoiding consideration of why people make such choices, a proper understanding is impossible.

Among both my work and campaigning colleagues, theories abound about why I get depressed; theories that seem to me as exasperating as they are inaccurate. The most popular is the 'working too hard' theory: 'You've been working too hard.' 'Are you sure your job isn't too much for you?' These theories often have a 'now you've got your come-uppance' feel to them. There have been people who resented my promotions, resented my publications, resented the conferences at which I was invited to speak, resented my capacity for work, finding good reason why they were right all along and I was wrong. I am completely unable to accept any of these 'working too hard' arguments: they simply did not fit with the pattern of my life. I have always worked very hard, both at my day job and outside, and I can see no relationship between the amount of work I do and the episodes of depression I experience. I might add that those who are closest to me know that I thrive on hard work, and have never believed such theories about my difficulties.

However, the 'working too hard' theory has had significant implications for my work. It was espoused by my head of department and by the occupational health physician, both of whom could exercise some control over whether I was allowed to return to work. The period that I was off sick (nearly six months) after my first diagnosis was artificially lengthened by this stance. On subsequent occasions I learned my lesson. I avoided going to occupational health and negotiated my return to work directly with my psychiatrist and manager. I have never since taken more than two months off sick, and with no noticeable detrimental effects. Indeed, it is easier to go back after two months than after six months: there is less to catch up on and my confidence is less eroded.

But at the bottom line I like a life that is full of varied things to do. I have always had an enormous amount of energy – more than most people I know. I am a quick worker and I love to work hard. I love the commitment, enthusiasm, engagement. I now see these qualities as a wonderful bonus of my manic depression. I do not believe them to be a cause of my depression but, if they are, I am prepared to take the risk. If getting depressed is the cost of living my life as I want to, then so be it. I can largely control my debilitating depressions with drugs, and if they get too bad then I know that ECT helps quickly.

I realize that not everyone shares my opinions, but I believe that there is something about the neurochemicals in my brain which means that most of the time they work really well and just occasionally they go wrong. I do not believe it is possible to know precisely why this might be. I am sure that many events in the external and internal environment can influence the action of such chemicals but I am reluctant to rule out notions of some form of 'genetic predispositions'. There is a lot of rubbish talked about genes. Genes do not determine what a person is like, rather they determine the characteristics with which we are conceived. There is then an ongoing reciprocal interaction between these characteristics and the social, political and material environment in which we live. It is this interactive process – the person acting on the environment and the environment acting on them – that I believe determines how a person will be. To assume some genetic or organic contribution is not to be determinist. It is simply one of many variables that influence the complex array of human behaviour and experience.

Power and Influence

There have been some who have seen my madness as a reason to doubt my capacities as a service provider and campaigner/writer and have used it to devalue what I say. I gave one talk that was written up in the local mental health network newsletter. Unfortunately, the reporter failed to record anything that I had said. Instead he described how the audience had difficulty in getting their heads around the fact that I was both a clinical director and a service user. Reactions such as this apart, it is undoubtedly the case that my multiple roles can also give me greater influence than someone who is not also a senior professional.

I frequently write and give talks about the nature of mental health problems and the way mental health services should be. Often I am asked to speak as a senior professional: someone who is basically a bit radical but clearly within the 'establishment' camp. In such instances my personal experiences of mental health problems can be used to challenge people's 'them and us' assumptions (and have certainly informed what I say). However, there are an increasing number of occasions when I am asked to give 'the user perspective' (as if there were such a unitary viewpoint). I am a kind of safe, not-too-threatening, user: one of 'us' really, who just happens, as an aside, to be one of 'them'. In such instances I suspect people are really not interested in hearing what those who use their services actually have to say; instead they want to feel as if they have listened by receiving a sanitized 'professional' account. I hope that I am sometimes successful in disappointing them, but I am afraid that people generally hear what they wish to hear and disregard the rest. My publications and senior professional status can get me a platform that I might not be permitted if I were solely a recipient of services, but this does not guarantee an independent user/survivor perspective. I cannot so easily divorce the various facets of myself and my relationship with mental health services. Neither can my audiences.

I think it is incumbent upon me to accept that my views about madness and services may have greater weight in various quarters because of my multiple roles. When I espouse a particular view or perspective it carries the weight of professional status, the credibility of my campaigning and writing and the expertise I have gained from living with my own madness and using services. While I am under no illusions about the limits of my influence, I think it is equally important not to underestimate the power of such a position. There are people who read what I write, listen to what I say. Even when they disagree, many take it seriously in a way that they might not but for my privileged status. As with any power, it can be used for good or ill. It is vital that my own views and decisions are not used to silence the equally important and valid perspectives of others. It would be wrong if my beliefs about the nature of madness or my decisions about treatment were imposed upon others as if they bore some spurious validity born not only of professional expertise but of personal experience as well. However, it would also be wrong for my perspective and experience to be discounted simply because I work within services and lack the faith in alternative therapies so popular in some quarters.

A Final Note on Choices

I have chosen to be 'out' about my madness. To talk about it and write about it openly. There were other possibilities. Since speaking of my madness I have communicated with numerous other mental health professionals who have also experienced mental health problems. People who, for fear of losing jobs, friends, careers, have chosen to remain very quiet about their experiences. Perhaps my decision to be open was taken from a position of privilege. I was already in an influential position in my profession and secure in a job where I believe I am a valued employee. However, in the present climate few jobs are that safe and discrimination against people who experience mental health problems is as rife as ever. Several concerned colleagues suggested that I keep quiet, if necessary talk about 'stress'. Why, then, did I choose to disregard this advice?

The short answer is that I had to. I have never found closets a very comfortable place to be. I find the deception and lying that they necessarily entail both difficult and dishonourable. I also hate the idea of people gossiping about my madness behind my back: if it is to be a topic of discussion then I want this to be out in the open where I can hear it, participate, correct misapprehensions. Most importantly, I work in a mental health service. I could see no way of keeping quiet about my own madness while providing a service for people with mental health problems. What would this say about the way I viewed those with whom I worked? What would it say about the 'them and us' divide, which blights mental health services?

I have chosen to speak openly about my madness, and I have also chosen to continue to work in mainstream mental services. While it is typically colleagues who ask about the former decision, other recipients of services and campaigners have questioned the latter decision. How can I continue to work in services which do so much harm to people with mental health problems in general, and women with such difficulties in particular? There are a variety of reasons.

I believe that, as long as most people use mainstream mental health services, it is my duty to work to improve them and make them more responsive to the views and wishes of those who need them. I am also very unhappy about the development of alternative therapies and facilities in what is essentially the private sector. However sliding the payment scale, any fees at all will be beyond the resources of many people who need help and I find it unethical that support and treatment be contingent on ability to pay. If help and support of all kinds are to be available to everyone who needs them, then changes must occur within the public sector, real changes that offer a greater range of assistance in a respectful manner and in accordance with the preferences of the person who needs them. Changes will be slow, too slow, but I have to believe that they really can happen.

Note

For further information concerning the Women and Mental Health Network UK, contact 15 Woodbury Street, London SW17 9RP.

References

Coward R (1989) The Whole Truth: The Myth of Alternative Health. London: Faber & Faber.

Jamison KR (1995) An Unquiet Mind. New York: Knopf.

Kitzinger C, Perkins RE (1993) Changing Our Minds: Lesbian Feminism and Psychology. London: Onlywomen Press, and New York: New York University Press.

Perkins RE (1991) Therapy for Lesbians: the Case against Feminism and Psychology, 2, 7–25. [Reprinted in Journal of Lesbian Studies 1997, 1: 257–271 and Rothblum ED (Ed) (1997) Classics in Lesbian Studies. New York: Harrington Park Press.]

Perkins RE (1994) Choosing ECT. Feminism and Psychology 4: 623–627.
  [Reprinted in Read J, Reynolds J (Eds) (1996) Speaking Our Minds. Milton
  Keynes: Open University Press.]
Perkins RE, Repper JM (1996) Working Alongside People with Long-term Mental
  Health Problems. Cheltenham: Stanley Thornes.
Webb J (1997) Review of 'Working Alongside People with Long Term Mental
  Health Problems' by RE Perkins and JM Repper. Self & Society 25: 52–53.

Chapter 10
Que Serà Serà

ROSE SNOW

Editorial

The terms madness and spirituality have been used liberally throughout this book, by the contributors and ourselves. For some of us, madness remains the most appropriate way of describing more extreme forms of mental distress – a paradoxically human alternative to framing such experiences as mental illness or disorder, even if no less pathologizing. We have assumed that for many, although not all, such experiences can have a spiritual dimension, or outcome.

Rose Snow is not only uncomfortable with the way unusual experiences are automatically construed by psychiatry as madness, but also has a very specific understanding of the nature of her spiritual experience. Despite being detained as a psychiatric patient, Rose believes that she was the victim of a series of misunderstandings, not least a failure to understand the complex nature of what was happening within her, in her spiritual realm. In her story, Rose introduces a quite different notion of spirituality to the consideration of the experiences commonly called madness. In her view, some people are involved in a special kind of emergence, which is different from the experience of consensual reality, and which can easily be mistaken for madness. Her vivid account of the journey through the tribulations of misdiagnosis, and what she considered to be wrongful imprisonment, is a powerful narrative indeed. An important question that emerges from Rose Snow's account is 'how do we distinguish the experience of madness from spiritual emergence?'. Indeed, we wonder if perhaps everyone who 'goes' mad is, in the strictest sense, emerging from one reality into another.

Rose Snow's account is significant on many levels, not least because it introduces, formally, into our discussion, the complex but specific idea of spiritual emergence. Like the psychiatric survivor movement, which has spread worldwide from Britain and the USA over the past 25 years, spiritual emergence is now being addressed not as a singular or extraordinary experience, but as an experience that may be open to everyone. This is not simply a new spin on the old idea of finding sanity in madness. Rather, it is an appreciation of the complex levels of human experience which, people like Rose Snow discover, extends into the Oneness that unites us all.

★   ★   ★   ★   ★

At the time of my first contact with psychiatry I believed I was a victim of misdiagnosis, imprisonment and torture. Eight years later I have not changed that opinion.

'Madness' is often projected by a society that fears change and difference on to individuals who are vulnerable to such projections, people who may be particularly sensitive to emotional undercurrents or receptive to ways of experiencing outside the norm.

I fear laying my words on the table. You may see only black ink and not the heart behind it, breaking out from constricted and shrunken psychic boundaries, into cosmic consciousness.

I was in the deepest grief; a loved one was newly dead.

What do I long for
     in forbidden memory of you?
What delicate field of love
     does this thick veil of tears protect?
I feel that you never were yet always will be.
What can make audible to me
     the separated silence of my grief?
What bridge to reality could form
     in the mist of this lunar landscape
And restore you soft in my heart?

Like the Tao I know you can not be named,
     nor contained, held still – even as a memory.
You live in my distant longing
     ever trying to picture you.
Knowing you too vast to picture
     I have nothing to comfort me.
Knowing you have always resided
     beyond my own dreams
I can not remember you.

A baby's unfolding trembling hand was his.
The ear that listened to those
      cold bitter and sullen in their grief was his

The back that carried so many
      broken across the water was his.
The colour that gave birth to all colour was his.

Time burns the crystal of my heart
      petrified when lost love dared
            look over its own shoulder..
                  lightens the song of my soul.

Can't describe him..
Can't miss him..
Can't remember him..
But as a hand moving slow motion across ultra violet light.

The first thing I saw as I was brought into the acute ward was a tiny woman in a sari walking in a circle, her hands joined in prayer. Her eyes had rolled and only the whites were showing. To my fragile perceptions she was a ghoul. I looked around and saw another tortured face – I believed I had died and gone to Hell. Shortly after that I collapsed into unconsciousness.

I don't remember being carried to the bed. I do recall seeing the closed curtains around the bed opposite me, like cubicles in a casualty ward. 'This is a trauma ward', I said to the nurse. My body was in trauma. I felt so badly hurt, like my skin was screaming, like a million nerves were exposed, and I was paralysed within it.

The nurse was kind, he held my hand. The physical contact was soothing and assuaged my fear. Eventually I was able to have some tea and toast, accompanied by a cocktail of drugs. The drugs made me talk a lot. I remember saying 'these are talking drugs'. I asked for pens and paper and wrote the names of people I loved and cared for and whom I thought 'good' on one side, and the names of people who were behaving badly and whom I thought 'bad' on the other. A couple of names remained in the middle as I was unsure about them. They took them away; I felt robbed. Before long I fell asleep.

When I woke up I was in distress and could not hold on to consciousness. Two strange men were sitting by my bed reading to me. I couldn't focus and could hear only an odd word at a time. Then I would slip into unconsciousness and come to again, to hear another few words. The men were looking intently at me. Sometimes I could see their lips moving but not hear the words. I was so frightened. I heard one of them say 'section...' I slipped into unconsciousness again.

I woke up terrified in the night. I held on to the sides of the bed, felt this great force pushing from underneath with an intensity capable of blowing me into space. My body arched and my hands hurt from gripping. The force felt evil.

The unreliable one had told me that they were planning to put a curse in his coffin. I felt I was dying with him.

I was a white woman aged forty-one, a wife and mother. I'd come home in distress after his funeral meeting, crying 'I'd rather crawl in the coffin with him, and let my body turn to worms, than let those bastards bury him'. He was old, very old, a traditional African. I adored him, like a father, and in the ten days since his death I had come to know for certain that he was an exceptionally gifted man. I clung to that bed like one whose life depended on it. I felt raped by evil and fought for my life. Terror racked my body and mind, rocked my spirit. I tried to pray, but I had trouble remembering the Lord's Prayer. I panicked and left the bed.

The ward was in semi-darkness and the night nurse sat knitting.

'Please help me', I said. 'I need to remember the Lord's Prayer, and I keep getting the lines mixed up. I believe those who worship the dark forces reverse the beginning and end of the prayer.'
'I hope *you* don't do that', she said, scoldingly, resuming knitting.

I joined my hands in prayer and began to pace up and down, my desperate spirit reaching out to recall the words. After an enormous effort to focus I eventually remembered it, the achievement pulling back together the shattered components of my self. I noticed that I was still wearing the pleated skirt and blouse from the evening before. They were crumpled. I wondered why they had allowed me to sleep in them. I felt dirty. In the morning I was given a hospital nightdress to wear that was split right up the back; so degrading. Much later, after I left hospital, someone told me that the 'being blown away' symptoms I experienced were known side-effects of the drug I'd been given.

Things had gone from bad to terrible in the ten days since Baba had died. He had been my music teacher. I had stopped lessons once when my second child was fourteen months, because it got too difficult. I used to play the drum with the child in a pouch on my back and carry both the child and the conga drum on the bus. The baby started to climb out when I was playing and the rehearsal room wasn't safe to let him roam around.

After a year I felt a huge gap in my life and went back to lessons. When I got to Baba's house he jumped up and danced for joy, repeating 'Rosie's come back, Rosie's come back'. He went to the phone and told an important person he must come immediately to greet me. The guy came. He danced with me and the old man put money on my forehead like they do to honour dancers in his own land. After that I saw him about twice a week, for years. I often used to say jokingly to my husband and friends, 'When that old man dies I'm going to crack up'. Little did I know...

It was Saturday morning and I was having a lie-in when the phone went. 'Baba's in hospital, it's bad... heart failure.' I threw on some clothes and drove to the hospital. He had an oxygen mask on and was wired up to a machine and kept his eyes closed. The doctor said she didn't know whether he'd pull through. I drove to find my drumming partner, told him to go quickly, that the old man might die.

I went home to my family. We were due to stay with relatives, leaving at lunchtime. I stayed behind, saying I'd join them later. I changed into colourful clothes, tried to be striking. I wanted him to notice me. At the hospital I bought flowers and a card. I wrote 'Baba, I love you, please don't die'. As I approached his bedside, his arms jerked up in spasm and he died. He was a hundred and three years old.

Someone I knew was there and we sat on each side of the bed, each holding one of his hands, communing with him. Then I heard yelling and was brutally dragged away from him and thrown to the end of the bed. The man was in huge distress and sobbing. He deeply embraced the dead body. A lot of people were standing at the foot of the bed and more and more people were arriving. Strong arms beckoned to comfort me but they felt untrustworthy and I ran away.

Away from the hospital, in our community, strange things started happening. There was talk of corruption, protection rackets, black magic, hidden treasure, wild fears, all of which was outrageous. I was a down-to-earth Taurean, in deep grief, with a responsible full-time job and a family to care for. I had an absolutely ordinary relationship with Baba, and had only recently been helping to arrange a Social Services attendance allowance for him. He was an ordinary, good man, a brilliant musician and teacher, a gentle and kind elder.

But now I could feel his spirit so strongly, and it felt different... so *powerful*. On one occasion I phoned a man staying at Baba's house, asking him to place a lighted candle where Baba had laid his head. The bed had gone, so the man put a night-light on the floor. When I arrived the next morning, the man was agitated, saying 'look!'. The night-light had burned four perfect, empty circles through a thick rug, a fitted carpet underneath, and linoleum underneath that. It had charred the floorboard itself, leaving a deep, charcoal-black circle on the wood. Nothing messy, just perfect circles. Someone put his carved walking stick in the hole, leaning against the wall. I could see it vibrating. The atmosphere was electric.

I sat beside this space with Baba's bible in my hands. The room felt blessed. I could hear energy buzzing all around me. I believe I received automatic writing. I copy from the original diary I wrote into at that moment:

> Lest you forget. You see Rosie and me, we're swinging. A candle you lit for me, you were baptised into the Catholic church which you loved so well, and now I am writing to you to show you how magnificent and glorious Love is.

Then the writing becomes faint, getting smaller and smaller as its trails down the page and circles round until it becomes indecipherable. It ends 'I am travelling far, there is great light and joy there'.

'Love knows not its own depth until the moment of separation.' The poet Kahlil Gibran's words rang terribly true. Grief grabbed me like a monster from the deep and sucked me into the depths. That night my inner or *third* eye opened wide. I could see Africa to my right and South America to my left and felt that my heart stretched round the world. I felt deep compassion and love and heard the voices of the ancestors begin to swell. I remember feeling terrified and calming them with my peace. I felt such love for humanity that my heart felt to be bleeding. My inner voice said '*You can heal*'.

What was happening? I wasn't prone to flights of fancy. I'd been a television stage manager for fifteen years, and now I was running a business and had several staff to manage. My husband was composing music and had taken two years off, and I'd been running the business on my own, with minimal help from him.

Things were getting difficult. My grief would cause me to burst into tears without warning. I was very tired.

Sometime around then, I had a gruelling but successful five-hour session with someone from the Inland Revenue, the upshot of which was an agreement that I owed no further tax. After the taxman went, the phone rang. It was someone from the same tribe as Baba, who said I had an important part to play in the burial ceremony, as I was so close and dear to him. After the phone call I went upstairs to my office and sat at my desk, my head on the table, resting in my arms. I entered a non-ordinary state of consciousness. My inner voice said '*The only way to say goodbye to a holy man is to kiss him goodbye*. The words were deep and sinister. I did not understand the implications, or realize what danger I would be in. There was to be a meeting in public rooms to arrange the old man's funeral. About a hundred and fifty people turned up. The atmosphere was awful. We were told there would be another meeting and none of us need attend, which some people argued about.

The old man was steeped in culture and his tradition was full of rituals rich in creativity and purity. I was brought up as a Catholic and spent my schooldays in a walled convent, draped in a white veil for mass most mornings. I too was steeped in ritual. In this time of fear and grief I found it natural to enact protection rites around my house and family. I performed prayers at strategic positions around buildings that our family used. Sometimes the children joined me in praying, and the prayers ran deep as blood.

The strife and paranoia in the community were almost palpable. In my fear, my faith wavered. One day I felt so threatened, I walked out and stood on the pavement calling to God in silence from the depths of my being. Said I, snapping my fingers: 'God if I have your protection I *demand* to see it now!' That moment, and out of the blue, several police cars converged from all directions, screeching to a halt simultaneously in front of me, parking all over the road. The drivers got out looking and sounding confused, as if they didn't know why they were there, or what they were looking for. I counted the panda cars. There were eight. They drove away after trying to sort things out through their radios. OK, God!

I was increasingly in awe of the power of the gentle man I was grieving for. I felt compelled to make sacrifices. My sacrifice would be that I could neither carry money nor spend money on anything. I had to practise humility. If I wanted cigarettes I had to beg for them on the street. I wasn't sleeping much. I seemed to have a never-ending amount of work to do. I typed Baba's obituary well into the night on one occasion. I had arranged for it to be submitted to a major newspaper for publication. He had, after all, been a notable musician. I was also trying to arrange for his funeral to be televised for local programmes and was typing things related to that. It was going to be a huge affair, with a float and musicians.

I was terrified of going to the second funeral meeting, but felt compelled to be there. A friend came to me, crying 'Rose, they've put voodoo on you'.

'Rubbish', I said. 'The only magic I believe in is the magic of Love.'

And I went. I got home at about three in the morning, after a horrible meeting, crying 'I'd rather crawl into his coffin and let my body turn to worms, than let those bastards bury him.' Which, as I said, is when my husband finally called the doctor.

There was little empathy between myself and my husband at that time. Our marriage was on the rocks. External events were making things worse and we were both under a great deal of stress, which was affecting our behaviour. In the few days before the meeting, I had developed the ability to speak in a language belonging to a higher plane of consciousness. I used this language on the duty doctor, thinking he would be an intelligent chap and understand. I had a touching faith in professionals, according to my adopted mother.

I was admitted to hospital about eight hours after the doctor called, having been further deprived of sleep. I was supported on both sides by my husband and his mother, as I could not walk. I was taken into a tiny room without windows. A female psychiatrist came in. She demanded of my tormented mind that I explain my family tree. They'd done that in casualty as well. How stupid, couldn't they see the state I was in?

She asked if I heard voices. I only ever heard my own inner voice, and, knowing that was not quite what she meant, I said no. She meant well though, and asked me what I would like.

'To lie under the trees, the tree spirits will heal me', I told her.

They took me into a dormitory and showed me a metal bed turned on its side with no mattress, which terrified me, so they took me out. My husband and his mother were still helping me stand up. I was dazed and staggering down the corridor. Next they took me into a big room with tables and chairs. My husband sat down and I sat on his lap with my arms around his neck and my head on his shoulder. I felt very confused and asked where I was. He told me I was in hospital.

'It's only made to look like a hospital', I said. 'It isn't really, there aren't any patients here, only staff.'

I was convinced that I had been captured, and that I was inside something evil. A nurse smiled at me, but it didn't feel genuine. I felt controlled by it. I stood up and saw the woman in the sari, whose eyes had rolled, walking towards me. It was due to the drugs I suppose, but I didn't know that and it terrified me. I ran down the corridor screaming and threw myself on the floor, either falling asleep or becoming unconscious.

Two days later, somewhat restored, I made friends with the patients and felt full of love for everyone. I had my first meeting with the consultant on the fourth day.

'I'm a Taurean', I said. 'One of the most balanced people you'll ever meet. I've had a rough time, but I'm all right now.'

I had been on an observation section, which he agreed to lift immediately. I was relieved, and phoned a friend. She told me that Baba's funeral was that lunchtime, that it would be all right to go, the hostility and malice had receded. A nurse wanted to go with me.

Everyone would be dressed in their most glorious clothes to honour this man. Once at home, I took from my wardrobe a ground-length, black, silk-velvet coat, flounced in twenties style, and a long silk-chiffon dress. I twisted my long hair into a tall knot on the top of my head, and I quickly wound it with a bright-blue silk scarf. I felt like a princess joining my 'chauffeur and lady-in-waiting' (a taxi driver and nurse). I called at our workplace, which was nearby, to pick up a poem that I had written to be read at the funeral by the child who had inspired it. My husband told me my desk had been cleared and the poem had been thrown away. I shouted and slammed the door. We missed the funeral cortege and burial by ten minutes.

When I got back to the hospital, the staff caught me coming in the door and read another section to me. They'd only just lifted the previous one. This place was insane. I was frightened. The nurses told me the consultant was applying for a treatment section: six months. I was called to an interview with him and felt fearful for my survival. I complained that all my power had been taken from me. I told him my life was full of love. He told me I was seriously ill. His words cut me like an axe.

A social worker came, whom I had not met before. She was cross with the consultant, and told me she had demanded that my GP visit me. She said they couldn't impose a treatment section until I had seen my GP; however, while I appeared a capable woman, the weight of the consultant's opinion was too strong for her to challenge effectively. I was led to a tiny room in a very dejected state. The consultant and a doctor from my GP's practice sat on a ledge with their legs swinging. I was told to sit in an armchair. They towered above me. Only the consultant spoke... 'Psychotic, manic depressive, seriously ill'. He was sectioning me for six months and telling me they could forcibly medicate me. I was terrified and told them that I was extremely sensitive to drugs and that most of them didn't agree with me. The GP sat there, silent like a puppet. Everyone seemed subordinate to the consultant. I was still terrified.

An old friend, a colleague from television days, visited me and, in despair, I pleaded with her to call Amnesty International. She looked harrowed. A nurse said the sectioning procedure had been 'messy'. She said the psychiatrist was in a bad mood. I telephoned the chief adminis-trator of the hospital and complained. A senior manager visited me. I was distressed and may have been incoherent. He asked if I had any complaints about the nurses.

'No, just the consultant', I said.

I heard no more about it.

It was my second week in hospital. The rug had been pulled from under my feet when I was diagnosed mad. I felt 'skinned', as if my ego had been ripped away. Now my spirit felt near death. I couldn't feel my body or mind, or any emotion, save the silent screaming for God. Then it happened. I was projected into the centre of the world process. There was a sacred combat going on between the forces of light and dark, and the resolution depended on the purification of my own heart. How my heart responded was vital. I felt crucified and seemed to face death. I knew I was playing a part in some incarnated mythology. Baba's words came back, lucidly to me: 'The world is a stage – we must each play our part.' I was obsessed by the meaning of the circle. I remembered Baba's words: 'Rhythm is round', he had drummed into us over the years, and 'Look to the front, the back, the left and the right, 360 degrees'. I thought of the four circles that appeared where his head had laid.

To balance such exalted preoccupations, I practised humility. Standing in the queue for the dinner trolley, I felt like a spiritual, social and political prisoner. I rejected any notion of illness, and took the degradation as an honour. I was also afraid I was being sacrificed. The consultant called me to interview. I sat waiting for him in an empty room. He did not turn up but sent a male student, whom I recall asking me about my sexual history.

The consultant called a case conference. I would have fifteen minutes to plea my case, as I saw it. I put on a business suit and prepared for my 'slot'. I was taken by taxi to another hospital and shown to a chair in a corridor where I remained alone for about an hour and a half. After a chorus of laughter sounded from a room nearby, a junior doctor emerged. I felt convinced they had already made their decision. I was now to have an interview of only five minutes. My heart sank further. I was led into the room where two leather armchairs faced each other. An old professor sat opposite me, and started to speak to me in a very affected way, as if someone had said '*Cue!*' There was no personal recognition. It was like a television interview. There was a one-way glass to our right. I could not see the onlookers. I felt intimidated by the professor's questions. Whatever I said in response seemed to show me in a poor light. I showed weavings I had made in hospital, which were highly intricate, to prove that I could concentrate and focus on reality. Later, I saw about thirty people pile out of the room where the interview had been viewed. I knew only two or three of them. I felt stitched up and scared for my survival.

My husband told me that if I ever wanted to get out I should stop challenging them and comply. I did, and before I knew it there was another, smaller case conference, to discuss my release. Everyone seemed cheerful. My husband and the consultant strolled down the corridor discussing music (the consultant was one of our business customers). I followed behind, wearing a big hat. From start to finish I was in hospital for five weeks.

By the time I got home I was a nervous wreck, as a result of the treatment and social humiliation. My husband said I couldn't work in the family business any longer as I couldn't take pressure. I kept to myself and stayed in the house. I was very fragile and my body would shake. I was told to see the disablement resettlement officer. I went in shaking and hardly able to speak, fighting the tears back. My heart broke with each word:

> I know I must *look* mad but I am not, I have been abused and held prisoner against my will.

Eight months after my release from hospital I was in the garden in the blazing sun. It was little, the surrounding walls whitewashed and the plants growing against them bursting with colour. I looked to the blue sky and my heart leapt. I thought of Baba and felt blessed to have known him. I wrote this poem and called it *Wild Wind*:

> These tears of searing pain
> Are at the same time
> Jewels of surging joy.
> The sparkle of dew
> On soft grass
> Can look as cold
> As a cutting edge.
> In death life exposes

Its deeper meaning.
In this white washed garden
Of lucid solitude
I feel you closer than ever.
And faith rides full sail high
On this wild wind of change,
Which I pray is whirling
Around your travelling light
In extravagant farewell,
And will know its own way home.

Minutes later, I was tending the flowers when a rush of energy shot from the base of my spine to my head, like a rocket. As I turned, I saw astral beings and life in every molecule of the air. That evening, after the children went to bed, I sat in an armchair by the log fire. I entered a state of non-ordinary consciousness and was for about two hours absorbed in total ecstasy, culminating in a vision of Mahatma Gandhi.

This altered condition lasted six weeks. I had taken acid (LSD) once in the 1970s and in many ways this experience was like a six-week 'trip'. It was extremely challenging, but I managed to integrate it well. I continued to look after the children and care for the house and garden, although I dropped unnecessary duties. At times it was frightening. I didn't know what was happening to me, the lucidity was so intense.

I was kneeling on the pavement tying the lace on my son's roller skate one day, when I decided I'd had enough. I got tired and cried and confided in my husband. He was afraid I was going mad. He urged me to talk to the consultant. I did – on my next visit I told him of the vision I had had of Mahatma Gandhi.

One day when the children were at school I felt an urge to tell my story properly. The need to be heard was as compelling as the need to give birth when the time comes. I drove to the ward where I was previously held, taking some blue Singapore orchids for the consultant as a peace offering. Naivety can be the death of innocence.

It was a sunny day and we talked in the garden, at my request. We sat opposite each other, cross-legged on the grass.

'I need to see an African psychiatrist. Is it possible?'
'No', he said.
'I need to tell my story, I feel it erupting like a volcano inside me.'
'You're starting another psychotic episode.'

I acknowledged that things were difficult, but said nothing would go out of control. I asked him again if I could see an African psychiatrist, as there was one working on the ward whom I had never spoken with. He hung his head. I asked him if I could confide in the head nurse, the African nurse whom I felt I could trust. He said no. I asked him if he had to do things 'by the book'. He nodded, looking utterly depressed. He asked me to wait while he went inside. He returned and said I should go straight to my GP to pick up a prescription. My heart was as heavy as lead.

In despair, I picked up the tablets from the chemist. I decided to go to the country for the weekend and took the little child with me, leaving my older son with my husband. I took the first tablet late on in the day. Shortly after I put my son to bed, I experienced a mental and emotional collapse akin to falling from the sky into a dark pit. I was curled up and crying like a baby. Momentarily I resided in a 'self' separate from this experience – my *being* – and I knew the drug was responsible for my pathetic condition.

I eventually climbed the stairs to the bedroom. I couldn't stand and clung to the window ledge, gasping for air. The sky was dark. My inner voice said *'If you can get through this night you will be able to help a lot of people'*. I saw the purple stars for the first time that night. They would sparkle, with each elevated thought. They were tiny and would shoot across my vision. It was magic, as if the stars were guiding me. Before long the struggle to remain standing was lost and I slid down, feeling poisoned in my stomach. I was afraid to call an ambulance as I feared my psychiatric label would prevent them looking at my physical symptoms that resulted from the drug. It was too risky: they'd think I was deluded, and drug me more.

I got to another room, where my symptoms worsened. My respiratory system became weak and a terrible crashing started in my head. My balance went and I was staggering. It went on for a long time. I remember trying to get out into the garden but I just couldn't manage the key. Soon, I collapsed. I scrawled a goodbye note and felt death approach.

I was lying at the bottom of the stairs. The horror that my little son would come down and find my body on the floor fanned a spark of life and gradually I felt some strength return. Eventually, I got up. I was still staggering and could not balance. The pain in my lungs, heart and head was terrible. I could not form a word to speak. I was crawling, devastated. I tuned into my internal energy or life force and I concentrated on expanding it until I perceived myself to be huge – much bigger than my body. Within this expanded landscape, the drug, which I visualized as an evil scorpion, played itself out like a firecracker – I felt it die. My symptoms had lasted fourteen hours.

I phoned the professor whom I felt had 'stitched me up' and told his secretary to tell him I believed he lacked humanity and that I would sue him. I said I thought he was a disgrace to the medical profession. I explained my symptoms to her and asked if there were an antidote.

Shortly after my phone call, my son came down the stairs, holding a fishing net.

'Mummy, you promised to take me fishing.'

We walked in silence for about five hundred yards to my favourite spot beside a stream in a secluded wood. On arrival, I was near collapse. I saw a man on the other side of the stream, elderly, with long white hair and a wide-brimmed straw hat.

'Can you help me before I fall into the water and drown?', I asked.

'I hope so', he said. 'I am a spiritual healer, a good witch.'

He ran to me, across the little bridge, and collected me in his arms. He sat me on a wall and held both of my hands. I cried for half an hour, he said, as though my very being was made of tears. Afterwards, I felt better and amazingly light.

My five-year-old stood with his fishing net in one hand and a box of magic tricks under his other arm.

'Thank you for making mummy better', he said.

'That little boy will be a great healer when he grows up', replied the man.

I told the man I did not want to forget him and asked for his address. We had no paper, but it was a simple address, which I never forgot. He became a treasured friend. The little boy is thirteen now. I do not know if he will be a great healer, but he has been commended for acting selflessly when he rescued a child who was trapped underwater in a canoeing accident.

Shortly after I got back to the house I heard from my husband and his family that I had to go to hospital or I would be taken in on section. I was taken back to the hospital against my will. On arrival I sat on the floor, leaning against the wall outside the office, as I could not stand. This time, the ward felt friendly. There were new staff from other cultures and I was met with smiles and warmth. I felt touched by magic and when I went on to the ward I sat beside a big man who had been agitated and threatening. He had stripped the walls of all pictures. There was phenomenal energy in the region of his head. I concentrated on drawing it down and he calmed.

He was gentle as a lamb with me, following me everywhere. The ward was touched by a still calm. The nurse had the most brilliant, genuine smile. She said she couldn't believe how beautiful the atmosphere was. I felt full of bliss.

The consultant arrived and I asked him if I could call him by his first name, so I'd be less frightened of him. He said yes. I felt ill and went to the bathroom. As I came back out, he approached me.

'You're high', he said.
'I'm not high', I said. 'I'm on my knees. You're the one who's high, high and fucking mighty.'

The nurses burst out laughing and he stormed off. I asked to see a general doctor because I thought I had experienced a heart attack. A doctor came, but didn't take a blood test. The examination was difficult as I couldn't sit up and didn't want her to lift me because she was pregnant. I had the bottle of drugs in my hand. I told her I'd had an allergic reaction to them. She took them away, but later came back and tried to give me the same drug again – chlorpromazine. Twice this happened. Both times I refused. Luckily, she accepted my refusal.

Days later, I ventured into the garden. I was tentatively walking down a tree-lined path, running alongside the geriatric wards, when I began to faint. The ward window was wide open and I managed to grasp the ledge as I fell. Only my head and forearms were visible to the three uniformed nurses inside. I looked, pleadingly, at them for what seemed like many torturous minutes, my mouth open but no sound coming out. I was fading and afraid I would die. They regarded me with puzzled suspicion. When I slipped down, four or five of them came rushing to help me. I was unable to lift a finger.

They put me in a wheelchair and took me back to the psychiatric ward. The nurse on duty was trained in general nursing and took my blood pressure. I noticed as he was tending me that his eyes were full of tears. I was not examined by a doctor. I couldn't sit up on my own and had to be helped out of bed. My son came and said 'you look really old, mummy'. Walking was difficult. I felt like a torture victim. My husband and brother lodged complaints about the drugs. In the day room I met one of the nurses who had been there during my first hospitalization, ten months before. She asked me what she could do for me.

'Give me a hug', I said.
She cried.

I spent just one week in hospital this time. My weight had dropped to under seven stone.

The following six months are blurred. I was washing up one day, when I thought *maybe you* have *gone mad Rose, have you ever considered that?* I went back to the psychiatrist. He now gave me lithium, saying I should probably have to take it for the rest of my life. I inhabited a lonely and hopeless space in my psyche, where darkness and fear ruled. After two months I came to the conclusion that *remaining in this space* was crazy, depressing and hopeless. *This* was madness. I sought out the healer who had helped me by the stream, for moral support and validation. He said saving me had made him feel like he had achieved an important part of his life's work. I felt humbled. I stopped taking lithium, but didn't tell a soul.

The ensuing few months were among the most difficult in my life. Our marriage was over. We flipped a coin to see who'd have the horrid job of petitioning for divorce. It turned out to be me. I fell ill, with excessive menstrual bleeding and abdominal pain. I felt my guts were being torn out. I knew the only way I could survive was to let my husband go with love. One time I looked into the mirror and saw his 'karmic reality'. The understanding came pictorially. His different past lives appeared in sequence, along with a vision of his present state of being. I was able thereafter to be more compassionate toward him, clearer as to what had happened between us.

The decree nisi came through and I moved house. In the car I couldn't bear it as we jolted and cornered. On arrival I was so weak I lay on the floor. I was cold and couldn't get warm. My eldest son, then thirteen, put lots of coats on top of me. The bedding was still packed away. I asked him to stay off school in case I needed him to call a doctor, because I couldn't have got to the phone. To my certain knowledge those two days were the only time one of my children missed school as a result of my ill health. I moved house alone with the children in February 1993, ill from the allergy, less than five months after my second hospitalization. If people really thought I was mad, why was I left alone with two children?

I saw a television programme about chlorpromazine that described my symptoms. There had been several deaths. I wrote to the consultant listing the adverse symptoms I had experienced, asking him to send the information to the Committee on Safety of Medicines. I sent a copy to my GP and sent both letters by recorded delivery. Neither of them replied to me. When I next saw the consultant, I asked for his response. He said he was pretty certain I had had an anxiety attack, not an allergy. I was appalled at his casual and callous attitude to what I knew to have been a serious physical situation.

I said 'I'm sure you didn't come into my life to torture me, but I must tell you that is how I have experienced your treatment'.

He replied 'I did not come into your life Rose. You came into mine.'

I felt desolate as I walked home through the park.

Later that month I got a letter from the consultant, saying he was changing his job and referring me to another hospital. I have not seen another psychiatrist (as a patient) since, nor have I taken any psychiatric drugs. That was seven years ago.

My main pain and outrage in relation to the experiences described is at how my sons were hurt, as children always are when their mothers suffer. The first year and a half alone with them was tough. Most times I couldn't look beyond the present. *'One step at a time, sweet Jesus'*, became my motto. In fact, I had to reduce my world to one *moment* at a time.

For over a year my inner voice had been telling me *'You can heal'*. Eventually, I phoned the National Federation of Spiritual Healers, who assigned tutors to me for a two-year training period, most of which I spent with one tutor, to whom I owe a lot. The first hands-on healing I did outside the training group was on a young African girl in torment. She said it was successful. The second was on a woman whose elbow had atrophied and locked from rheumatoid arthritis. The woman gasped as it gently released under my hand. I still wasn't well, and I was unable to earn a living any other way, so I went out cleaning twice a week. I did not resent it as I knew it would strengthen my character. In any event, I needed the money. My hospitalization had ruined my career, as well as my health. In November 1994, I gave up hands-on healing, on the recommendation of my current spiritual teacher.

On a beautiful afternoon in May 1993, I sat under blossoming trees, feeling in absolute unity with nature. I offered my life to God. That night I was projected into a waking nightmare. My bedroom filled with 'pressure' and seemed disconnected from the ordinary world. My eyes locked open and I was pinned to the bed, unable to move.

Outside, the most savage, unnatural pressured energy was on the verge of caving the windows in. I could 'see' it. It was enough to suck me into outer space. I was unable to move for hours. I was lying on my bed, on my back, my arms outstretched, as if I was on a crucifix. One wrong move or single negative thought and I was done for. The experience was savagely intense, and the terror I experienced was beyond words.

I recognized the voice of a mythological character from West African culture, the God of Thunder. I recalled how he was supposed to invoke unspeakable fear. He certainly roared for some time. I felt the bed shaking and when I looked I saw it vibrating. Strangely, I was not afraid of him. I knew he was not angry with me. I had been through so much already. My faith in God was strong and I felt innocent and helpless in the face of such great forces.

Nevertheless, the experience reached a stage where I felt I was being destroyed, at which point something firmly gripped my right hand. I gasped and looked to my right (my arm was still outstretched). I saw and felt a white hand, cool but not cold, strong and male. It held my hand. Holding his hand was another, and another holding that, and on and on. A chain of hands, white and light, extended out of the room, up into the sky, up into the universe, connected up to the 'royal' spirits, to the throne, my spiritual ancestry. I was safe. I had all that love and protection. I fell asleep in the same position in exhausted ecstasy.

When my sons woke me the following morning, I got washed and dressed as usual. I always had the boys to deal with. They were now thirteen and seven. I went out to bring in the washing from the garden. My heart sank when I saw the washing line was down, and the washing on the ground. There was no wind and it was warm, probably had been all night. The invisible 'pressure' must have brought the line down. Or maybe the line had just rotted. Who knows?

During the experiences I have described, a link with consensus reality always remained. I knew I had to stay in touch with the experience of the ordinary world and managed to do so. I guess the fear of the unknown and treatment by the psychiatric system, for some, makes this impossible in such circumstances. The interests of my boys, whom I loved deeply, felt so urgent to me that whatever I was going through I stayed true to my role as their mother. The experiences humbled me, as though I was being tested by God. It wasn't safe to share my experiences or fears with anybody. I knew I wasn't ill but didn't know how much more I could take. Oh, how I wanted to be ordinary.

The two years training with my tutor from the National Federation of Spiritual Healers concentrated on removing internal barriers and introduced subtle internal mechanisms to effect change. With increased self-understanding, I was able to transform much of my anger into something creative. Inspired by some of our recommended reading, I faced my internal monsters. Although those of us training together worked well as a group and I was able to make myself vulnerable by describing my experiences to an extent, I knew I still had not told 'my story'. I knew it would take a special kind of person to counsel me.

I met her in August 1994, two years after the second hospitalization. She was seventy, had a background in psychiatric social work and child guidance and was selling cards to raise money for the Coalition of Arab and Israeli Doctors. After five sessions, she appeared at my door, saying she could not continue to counsel me as she had become too fond of me, too emotionally involved. She said I could continue to have her heart, her mind and her 'ear', but not a professional relationship. She said this had never happened to her before. It was as though we rediscovered each other at this point as mother and daughter.

I was sitting at my desk shortly after meeting her when I perceived that something big was going on in my heart. It was painful, emotionally, physically and mentally. It felt like a tomb door opening. My creativity was freed and I wrote a poem which came out complete, and was dedicated to the consultant who 'dealt' with me, the first of some forty-one poems (my age when I was hospitalized) that I wrote within the next twelve months.

Whilst suffering illness for over two years from the allergy to chlorpromazine, I did without medical treatment. I believe attempts were made to shove my life-threatening, allergic reactions under the carpet. I had no money for private medicine and suffered near paranoia about allopathic doctors. It was so bad that if an ambulance passed me in the street my legs would shake and I would feel faint. During those difficult times, I relied on prayer. After two years some money became available and I paid for very effective treatment from a traditional Chinese doctor. My adopted mother too played an enormous part in my recovery, offering tremendous practical support. When my liver and spleen were bad and I didn't have the strength to walk down the road to fetch the children from school, she was there to help, as she was when I needed to rant and rave about the psychiatrist and the psychiatric treatment I suffered.

I began to trust allopathic doctors again after one came on a home visit a couple of years ago when my heart was playing up. I finally felt vindicated in wanting to reject any notion of 'mental illness' when, in 1995, I read *The Stormy Search for the Self* and then *Spiritual Emergency* by Cristina and Stan Grof. In these texts, and in *The Far Side Of Madness* by John Perry, I found leading research psychiatrists writing academic accounts of experiences just like mine, describing them as part of a unifying process that leads individuals to a higher state of personal development. Stan Grof has since then written a clinical diagnostic framework for Spiritual Emergence and Spiritual Emergency, a framework used by a growing number of British psychotherapists. I am developing training initiatives for clinicians with some of them now. Our presentations balance the theory and the experience of spiritual emergence and emergency.

I started doing informal research on the subject of spirituality and mental health in 1993 – it was one of the few things I could do at my own pace. I was still ill from the allergy. I then became inspired by the idea of Local Exchange Trading Schemes (LETS) in a mental health setting and founded LETS Make it Better in Manchester – a user-led project. Many people were involved, and a circle of goodwill around the city was exposed, inspiring many LETS in mental health settings to spring up in the region. The project was awarded a Certificate of Commendation from the North West Regional Health Authority in its Health Challenge awards for two years running, the latest one for our 'excellent work in improving health'. In 1997 I was employed by NW Mind to develop and facilitate a diverse cultural conference on the subject of spiritual emergence versus psychosis. It was a catalyst for positive change for many people. Now the task it to set up practical responses for people experiencing spiritual emergence. I am part of a working party set up by Central Manchester Healthcare Trust to look at spirituality and mental health. When I look back at how damaged I was by psychiatric intervention in my spiritual emergency and emergence over the two years I suffered it, I wonder if the person I have described above was really me. It doesn't seem so! I feel healed now, and in many ways I can't remember the period.

In June 1997, I went to a mental health training event and heard from an Australian mental health professional that, in the late 1980s, an extensive survey was done on conditions on an average acute psychiatric ward in Australia. He said one the findings was that around 34% of patients would have an additional diagnosis of post traumatic stress disorder, commonly diagnosed in survivors of car crashes, wars, disasters, etc. They were unsure whether the condition was due to trauma before, during, or after admission to the acute ward. This information was motivation to completely redesign admission to and treatment on acute wards throughout Australia.

I was the only 'survivor' at this training session, which had been staged for professionals. The morning session had been brilliant but very challenging for me, as it was given by another survivor/pioneer who struck a very deep note. By the time the Australian psychologist spoke I had a headache. After he presented the information about post-traumatic stress disorder, the headache got worse. By the time I got home, it was very bad. I lay on the living room floor and couldn't cope with anything. I screamed in pain. After a disturbed night, I awoke, shaking, exhausted and almost unable to move. My skin felt like it did after admission to hospital, as if all the nerves were exposed, and I was paralysed inside. A suppressed memory had risen to haunt me.

I spent two days in bed, out of action. I knew what was happening and felt resentful. When I lay in bed after the first admission, eight years ago, I had known I was in trauma, badly hurt. The Australian results seem to suggest this was more than likely to have been the case. I probably did have post-traumatic stress disorder. In late June 1997 the involuntary spontaneous re-enactment of it was almost as terrible. Although the completely inappropriate treatment I received in these circumstances left me thinking again about violation of human rights and litigation, I believe that, overall, I have grown as a result of my experience. My spiritual awareness has almost always given me solace and succour, no matter how wounded I felt. When it didn't, it was an opportunity for me to rebuild my faith. Truly, I am a happier, more talented person than I was before, with more hope. I know myself, I know why I'm on the planet. And I gained a mother and father, both amazing role models, after having lost my natural ones long ago in childhood. The boys and I have 'made it'. We're free from all sorts of oppression. My eldest is eighteen now; he's just climbed to Annapurna Base Camp in the Himalayas. I still see tiny purple stars every day. They wink at me or shoot across my vision. Sometimes, they ride on the scent of flowers. When I was washing up at an artist friend's house, several fell into the saucepan! I often hear enchanted music in the silence, sometimes very loudly. I can feel the 'silver thread' that connects me to the Source. It swings me and I hear it buzzing. Sometimes I feel empty, a great hole in my centre – like I'm at one with the universal flow and I exist outside time.

I think I was probably born with my third eye a bit open. I could see *through* the flowers when I was little and I played with the little people (fairies) when I was seven, on a hillside in southern Ireland. My heart was full of joy with my cousins, away from the roar of London. The little people could jump high. I remember being incredibly moved when I first saw them, saying 'Wow, they really do exist!'. We played hide and seek with them for hours and hours. It felt like magic at the time. I don't remember my aunt's exact words, when I told her, but she didn't believe me. I didn't pursue it and felt the dramatic invasion of a deep stabbing loneliness, which would haunt me for most of my life. We should tread with special care with the young, for when we project our poverty of knowledge on to them the results can be heartbreaking.

I had a dream a year before Baba died, a prophetic dream. We were walking arm in arm, when he turned to me, paused and said 'I'm going to die now'.

'We'd better find somewhere warm for you to lie down then', I replied, unperturbed.
I noticed a parade of shops ahead. One stood out, emanating a welcoming yellow glow, a dry cleaners.
'He needs to die now. Can he lie down on your floor as it is warm and clean here?' I asked.

'Yes', said the assistant, as she went away to get a plastic bag. I presumed the bag was to put the body in. Baba lay down and I knelt on the floor beside him, holding his left hand with my right hand. As he died, a fluid energy coursed from his arm through my hand and up my arm, like a river. It was very disturbing. Although it was invisible, I knew it was white. The woman came in again and I walked out of the door on to the pavement.

There was utter chaos, like in a hurricane. The air was thick with dust and rubble and planks of wood. Even trees were flying. All sense of direction was gone and it was impossible to identify landmarks. I woke up with a start, still feeling in grave danger, and drove straight to Baba's house, distressed, expecting to find him dead. I banged loudly, for some time, on the window. He woke up, quite gently, and smiled. He would not die for a year yet.

The dream had proved true. After Baba's death, a most dangerous chaos ruled in my life for three years. Knowledge that he was my father, my spiritual father, whom I was blessed to have encountered in my lifetime, was driven into my being so many times, so deeply, in so many ways, so that there could be confusion, no wondering, no lack of confidence.

Chinese and British scientists have proved the existence of a microscopic, white fluid energy system, running through the body.[7] The dry cleaning shop was an appropriate symbol. I was to be cleansed, purified. My experiences were deep and extreme, like the chasm ripped in the earth, when his energy departed.

To me, psychiatry seems like a '*flat earth*' approach to the psyche. While psychiatry might diagnose me thus and so, I would say this of my experience: I've sailed right round my mind and I *did not fall off*! Bereft, I drifted in darkness, through turmoil and fire, captured by a hostile tribe, half dead, in abject loneliness, through the long winter of my soul, with two

[7] Dr Kim Bong Han, University of Pyongyang in North Korea, has apparently, in discovering the existence of meridians, repeated the work of Sir Thomas Lewis in England (British Medical Journal, February,1937) who found an 'unknown nervous system, unrelated to the sensory or the sympathetic nervous systems'.

little children, seeking the light. And I found it.[8] Looking back, I know only too well that I was, at times, deeply disturbed. One manifestation of my disturbance was that I was unable to remember Baba. I just *couldn't* think of him. The poem 'Moving Slow Motion', which opened this chapter, was the result of the first time I dared remembered his gentleness, *three and a half years after his death*. Even my tears were afraid to fall.

If you want to make things better for people who get into the psychiatric system, remember to work with them from the perspective of their reality, as best you can. To impose a view of reality born of mechanistic models of the psyche and the soul on someone in torment is not intellectual freedom. It's about as free as a hand that's severed from the arm. I write this chapter for my ex-psychiatrist, who didn't enquire about my life.

Calling people 'mad' who explode taboos or discover new regions of the 'world' won't work in future, as the new tide carries waves of searching questions. The work is to forgive each other and forgive ourselves. But let us not fall into the trap of saying to someone who's been hurt, 'Forgive!', without knowing what forgiveness is. To forgive someone requires that we transform into love all the emotions we feel or felt as a result of being hurt or damaged. In cases of severe hurt, to say it is difficult is an understatement. One has to reclaim one's vulnerability, to become open and light and fully engaged again.

When I was on the way to forgiving, and I was feeling my pain and shedding my victimhood, I had to wrap myself in symbolic cotton wool, the agony was so extreme. The pain was sculpted into me – I had to unravel it and remodel myself. Transformation is an 'experience'. Never think true forgiveness is easy, nor underestimate its power. I don't have to like my ex-psychiatrist, and I don't. I do however, have to love him as I recognize him as a child of the universe and part of the true Oneness. If you read this, know that I believe you must be a karmic friend, you've helped me so much, freed me from oppression, got me on the right path. The anger I felt towards you inspired all of my current projects and made me a poet, and I've still got some left for something new. Que Serà Serà.

References

Gibran K (1992) The Prophet. Harmondsworth: Penguin.
Grof C, Grof S (1992) The Stormy Search for the Self: A Guide to Personal Growth Through Transformational Crisis. Los Angeles: JP Tarcher.
Grof S, Grof C (Eds) (1989) Spiritual Emergency: When Personal Transformation Becomes a Crisis (New Consciousness Reader). Los Angeles: JP Tarcher.
Perry JW (1990) The Far Side of Madness. New York: Spring Publishing.

---

[8] I must acknowledge my spiritual master Ching Hai Wu Shang Shih.

Chapter 11
The Medical Model and Harm

JUDI CHAMBERLIN

Editorial

Almost 150 years ago a first-hand account of recovery from madness was published in England. John Perceval, drawing on his own experience, believed that as much as a person in psychosis might be ill, he was also the victim of a human earthquake and was very much in need of help, in the same sense that all victims of natural disasters need help. For Perceval, that help was rooted in compassion. Acting on that belief he committed himself to the task of helping others– especially those with authority over the insane [sic] – to appreciate the central importance of compassion.

More than 20 years ago Judi Chamberlin emerged from her own human earthquake as the American successor to Perceval. She has developed over the past 25 years a powerful presence on the world psychiatric scene, becoming a provocative and challenging advocate for change. She has questioned not only the validity of the concept of mental illness but, more importantly, the value of the psychiatric responses to mental illness. Here, Judi reflects on her formative experience, describing the circumstances of her original collapse into profound depression, and how that experience brought her – painfully – to the brink of the understandings that were to fuel her subsequent advocacy work.

Judi Chamberlin shares with Dan Fisher a belief in the civil rights status of the struggle for empowerment of people with experience of mental distress. Her work, with Dan and others at the National Empowerment Centre in Massachusetts, is the formalized outcome of her appreciation of the failings of psychiatric care and treatment, all those years ago. In this short essay she illustrates the painfulness of the experience of inappropriate help. In a perverse sense, we should be grateful that it was so poor and inappropriate, since it served as the stimulus for the establishment of a modern successor to John Perceval, the now worldwide psychiatric survivors movement.

* * * * *

'Mental illness' is a theoretical, medical explanation of people's distress. Those of us who deny the validity of the illness theory are often accused of ignoring people's suffering. Nothing could be further from the truth. In this chapter, I shall explore my own experiences of acute distress that have been labelled as 'madness' or 'mental illness' and illustrate how it is in fact medical theory that obscures people's ability to understand and deal with their own pain.

At the age of 21, after experiencing a miscarriage, I plunged into a depression so extreme that I was unable to function. I stayed in bed crying, day after day, not bathing, barely eating and unable to believe the fact that the baby was no longer within me, was not to be born. After a period of several weeks, my obstetrician, with whom I had an excellent relationship, became alarmed and referred me to a psychiatrist colleague. Thus began the medicalization of a real and painful experience, and its transformation into 'mental illness'.

Because I liked and trusted my obstetrician, I came to the psychiatrist with trust and hope. I knew I was filled with pain, and I believed that he could do something about it. If ever the stage were set for a positive therapeutic relationship, this was it. But, unbeknown to me (and perhaps even to the referring doctor), this psychiatrist was a firm believer in a strict medical approach to my suffering. Within the first ten minutes of our first interview, he opened a drawer of his desk, a drawer I could see was filled with samples of all kinds of pills, and selected a few for me. These pills, I was assured, would help me to feel better.

Looking back on it now, I am amazed that I accepted this offering so readily. But, in retrospect, it is not so surprising. I was young, I was trusting, I had no reason to doubt the expertise of the doctor, and I knew of no alternatives. In the mid-1960s there was little recognition of the real grieving that women experience in losing a pregnancy: the conventional wisdom was that it wasn't a *real* loss, like losing a full-term baby. There were no support groups, no confirmation that my pain was real and valid. There was only the unbearable suffering, and this offer of help. So I took the pills and wanted to believe they would help.

Moving my pain out of the realm of shared human (female) experience and into the realm of medicine and pathology was the first step in alienating me from my own feelings and my own power to heal myself. I went home, wept, took the pills, visited the doctor, wept, took the pills, and the awful days dragged on. As it became clear that the pills were not the answer, that I was not getting better, the 'logical' conclusion came easily: that I was truly and severely ill. Of course, the doctor did nothing to dispel this belief.

Hospitalization was the next step. Perhaps a few weeks earlier I would have rejected going to hospital; now, it seemed inevitable. The logic seemed clear and irrefutable: if I had an illness, and it wasn't getting better, obviously more intensive treatment was required. I entered the hospital (a psychiatric ward in a highly regarded general hospital) sure that here, at last, someone would know how to make me better.

The medicalization of human suffering continued. It seemed odd to me that no one on the staff seemed concerned with my feelings and opinions of what was wrong, yet it made perfect sense. After all, these were the experts, the ones who knew how to cure me. I so desperately wanted to believe that they knew something I didn't.

How different it would have been if I had found someone who regarded me as a full human being, filled with real human pain, rather than as a disease entity. Real help, I know now, would have consisted in acknowledging my suffering as real, and in guiding me toward ways of living with disappointment, rather than stamping out its existence with drugs. I know that now because, years later, I was helped in exactly that way.

This most recent time it was the loss of a love relationship that triggered an intense depression and the wish to die. But this time I had the services of a crisis centre that was non-medical, non-psychiatric, and which used the common humanity of the helpers and the helped as the mode of 'treatment'. This crisis centre was started and run by people who believed that even the most intense crises could be alleviated by a reaffirm-ation of shared humanity rather than the distancing of psychiatric labelling.

How profoundly different it was to find that my thoughts and beliefs were taken seriously, even when they were 'irrational'. I was encouraged to express my feelings, either verbally or through crying, screaming, or whatever else seemed appropriate to me. In the psychiatric system, such expressions of extreme emotion are seen, once again, as symptoms, and every effort is made to stop the person from expressing them, through drugs, isolation rooms and physical restraints. Here, instead, I was assured that I would be kept safe, and that the release that came with letting go would be ultimately healing.

I remember how, during the first episode, I became convinced that my pain had isolated me from the rest of the world to such an extent that I was lost in outer space, far from the earth that I knew was my home and longed to return to. I would scream as loudly as I could, in the hope that someone on earth would hear me and would guide me home. When I was drugged or secluded in response, the message was clear: it really was hopeless, I would never find my way back, I would die in the coldness and isolation of my exile from the world. The treatment only prolonged my suffering.

If the 'irrational' actions of the person in crisis have meaning, help must consist of providing places and ways for the individual to discover that meaning, and to find ways of living in a non-ideal world. But the psychiatric system, which ostensibly exists to help people, in fact has the social function of labelling and isolating people whose behaviour is disturbing to others and to the social order. Drugging, electroshock and similar methods are designed to quieten the sufferer and make him or her more socially acceptable. The pain may still be there, but the person in a drugged stupor is far easier for those around them to deal with.

It is important to point out that not everyone who ends up in the psychiatric system is in a state of emotional turmoil, as I was. People are subjected to the psychiatric system primarily because their behaviour is distressing to others, even when they themselves are not troubled by it. This is why it is important, in every discussion of reforming or transforming the psychiatric system, to be aware constantly that different people in the system need different things: a crisis centre would have been very helpful to me, for example, but it would not be a meaningful alternative for the individual who had been hospitalized because of an ongoing family conflict, and who simply wanted to be left alone.

During my journey through the psychiatric system, I was transformed, first, from a person who was suffering a real loss to a person whose grief was a 'symptom'. I then became a patient, a person who needed drugs to control the symptom, and who belonged in a hospital because of the degree and intensity of my illness. I then was further transformed into an involuntary patient, medically and legally assumed to be unable to define or act on my own best interests. By this time, the cause of the original pain had long since been forgotten by those who were diagnosing or treating me. I was simply a 'psychotic', a 'schizophrenic', someone whose beliefs and feelings did not matter. I was essentially an object to be processed through a system designed to control my behaviour and make me either socially acceptable enough to be released or simply another 'chronic patient'.

Hope and healing had no place in this scheme of things. In fact, what I saw, from the very first day in the very first hospital (there were to be six hospitalizations, ranging from short-term psychiatric wards to an end-of-the-line state psychiatric institution), was the vision of what I could easily become: a drugged, stuporous person who was defined (and who defined herself) as a diagnosis first, a person second. I met such people in every hospital I was in: we told each other our diagnoses before our names, a litany of what hospitals we had been in, what drugs we had taken, how many times we had attempted suicide. Thoughts of an independent life, away from doctors and hospitals, receded quickly and seemed more and more impossible.

Hospital practices reinforced this sense of hopelessness. It was constantly emphasized that the drugs we were given were as necessary as insulin for diabetics, that there was something wrong with us on an essential medical level. Even when it seemed clear to me that some of my fellow patients had lives that seemed guaranteed to drive anyone crazy, no one seemed to notice. And, since I was only a patient, taught to doubt my own perceptions, it was easy to convince myself that my perceptions were wrong, were just a further manifestation of the wrongness – the 'sickness' – of my thinking.

Being treated like an object quickly made me feel like one. Feeling like an object was said to be a 'symptom' of my 'mental illness'. Therefore, obviously, I was mentally ill. Struggling to make sense of my circumstances, I had been given a frame of reference that led inexorably to hopelessness and despair (further proof that I was suffering from an incurable illness).

At the same time, my 'wrong' thinking continued to hold out the only hope I had. I was angry – angry about being locked up, treated like an object, ignored, drugged. Although constantly told that my anger was a symptom, some part of me held on to it as a link to the person I had been, the person I wanted to become again. I could feel and, under the circumstances, anger seemed logical. When I let myself feel my anger, I felt more alive than I had felt in months. But every expression of anger brought more drugs, more 'treatment'. I felt trapped; I *was* trapped – for while all my instincts said to fight, it was made clear to me that I was expected to give up, to become passive, compliant, a 'good' patient.

Fortunately, I was not alone. Always, in every hospital, there were at least a few patients who refused to give in, and we sustained and supported one another. In one hospital, where I was abruptly taken off all medication, it was another patient who explained to me that the weird feelings I was experiencing were withdrawal symptoms, not 'psychosis'. In another hospital, it was a patient's advice not to be seen crying that taught me a valuable survival lesson: that being thought of as 'depressed' could have only negative consequences.

There was also the dream to sustain me, the fantasy that some day I would return, together with all the others who had been so beaten down, to free ourselves from the power of psychiatry and the walls and locked doors of institutions. I told no one about the dream – if being labelled 'depressed' was a risk, being called 'paranoid' would be an even bigger one. Yet alone in my bed at night, I would imagine armies of mental patients, battering down the gates, escorting the inhabitants safely to freedom, and blowing up and burning down the empty places of our incarceration. In the dream I was strong, and that feeling of power made me feel a little less helpless, a little less alone.

There was little support for my anger. When I expressed it, I was drugged or secluded. And it wasn't just within the mental health system that it was seen as illegitimate. I tried calling the American Civil Liberties Union and the Legal Aid Society when I was told I was being committed, asking for help in fighting for my freedom. But it seemed that freedom was not something that 'mental patients' deserved: neither agency expressed any interest in my case or my cause. In fact, I was told that if the doctors decided I needed to be in a state hospital, that surely was where I needed to be. It was clear that if I wanted to be free, I was going to have to fight for it alone.

The survival skill called 'playing the game' was another thing I learned from the patients around me. Playing the game meant learning how to give the *appearance* of being a 'good' patient. It meant 'co-operating' with treatment, 'volunteering' to make beds and mop floors and wash dishes, expressing appreciation for the 'help' and 'support' of the hospital. I thought of it as lying, but lying in the pursuit of a greater good. It was amazing how easily the staff accepted these lies. At times, I expected my transformation from troublemaker to 'good patient' to be greeted with at least a little scepticism, but it never was. Since I had been told that schizophrenics couldn't control their behaviour, the staff apparently believed it was impossible for me to be acting purposefully toward my goal of freedom.

I was left, alone and unsupported, to puzzle these things out for myself. All those things that were truly healing and sustaining had to be kept secret, making any real healing all the more difficult. The environment of the mental hospital promoted the very fragmentation that was, supposedly, the mark of my 'illness'. I felt alone, untrusting, wary of others – 'symptoms' all!

Mental hospitals, operating under the so-called medical model, can never be places of true healing. Patients *can* be controlled, and can learn to internalize those controls so that their behaviour appears more 'normal'. They can be drugged, and can learn to function under the influence of the drugs. But to allow people to experience their feelings, to express their pain, to grow and to heal is a far different enterprise, one that is about freedom, not control. And mental hospitals were not built to set people free.

Chapter 12
Conclusion

PHIL BARKER, PETER CAMPBELL AND BEN
DAVIDSON

The Human Progress Project

As we get set to launch into the new millennium, we could look back on the past century with wonder and amazement. In the past fifty years the Western world has swept through one amazing, pioneering adventure after another: from splitting the atom, and depositing a man on the moon, to the prospect of cloning new life. Science fiction has become scientific fact. The drive towards new technological frontiers that characterizes the end of the twentieth century leaves us, though, with a quandary – what, exactly, to make of it all. Here we sit, surrounded by 'smart drugs' to take away the drudgery of life; perhaps we are knee-deep in the litter of lottery tickets, hoping for an end to our material insecurity; and watching us, from our digital television sets, is Dolly the cloned sheep, an ominous presage of what biomedical advance might conjure up next.

Orwell and Huxley could be sitting with us, no doubt shaking their heads either in disbelief or resignation. If they were trying to warn the world, fifty years ago, rather than just writing novels, they would not be surprised that, despite our progress, we remain dissatisfied, even as we clasp our well-thumbed copy of the *Celestine Prophecy* or one or another manual of positive thinking.

There is always a message in misery. One narrative suggests that we feel doomed because we shall soon be humanly redundant: science will create a world where we no longer need to work, all our needs being met by the great god of technology; where loneliness too will disappear – if we have no relationships they will be created for us, virtually if necessary. The challenge of how to pay for it will, of course, remain. Perhaps our *fin de siècle* misery, not to say angst, suggests that the cost of the dream of progress is already gathering interest, with bankruptcy looming.

Out of Affluence – Misery

Depression, a psychic plague known only too well to the ancient Greeks two and a half millennia back, and never far from the minds of humanity, has excelled itself in the late twentieth century. It has finished second only to coronary heart disease in the list of the health care costs in the Western world. In the developing world it is gradually making progress, moving fast through the pack, standing about eighth, ready to launch a sprint to overtake hunger and all the physical ailments that depend on starvation for their success.

Ironically, the sheer ordinariness of depression means that we hardly talk about it, or at least not in fearful terms, often dismissing it as an ailment of the 'worried well', a mere neurosis, even when of truly epidemic proportions. Instead, we worry – or are encouraged to worry – about other forms of madness, and madmen and women. Mental health experts in the USA, Europe and the Antipodes ponder the rash of similar-looking catastrophes involving (allegedly) crazed gunmen (and occasionally gun-children) mowing down relative strangers, if no immediate family could be found. Psychosis – the good old-fashioned madness favoured by Hollywood producers – has come out of the run-down asylums to haunt the streets of community care. Images of madfolk cultivated in the tabloid press and the popular imagination suggest no difference between the typical person experiencing mental health problems and some (usually black) version of Alfred Hitchcock's anti-hero from the film *Psycho*.

Such images evidently serve an ideological function when seen in the light of the fact that most people continue to have considerably more to fear from their immediate family than from any madman (or woman) prematurely released from community care. Or, we might say, they have more to fear from ordinary problems of malice, greed and depression – whether individual or societal.

In any event, as we fret, in our isolation, about the threat posed by 'mad-axe-folk' living in hostels that are far too close for comfort, depression folds its dark wings around communities and societies that have lost their souls with the decline of popular religion, and look set to lose their hearts, as fellowship and true community succumb to the paranoid cyber-culture.

Madness in Context

A more honest assessment of our human progress – which might explain our current anomie – is that humanity has been seriously on the slide for

50 years. If we doubt this, we need only casually flick through our Western social statistics: in particular those for crime and poverty, as well as mental ill health. These three are probably siblings, one fostering the other incestuously. And then there is crime on a larger scale. As the last veterans of the First World War mark the 80th anniversary of its conclusion, entreating the world, for the last time they can, not to forget, Europe takes a last, long look at the havoc wreaked on the psyches of the Great War generation, and at the impact on generations that followed. Meanwhile, the whole world might do well to reflect on the cumulative effect on the psyche, the social world and the collective unconscious of this and also the Second World War, the Holocaust, the Cold War, Vietnam and latterly other adventures on the North–South divide. The ease with which the West, particularly America, has been able to replay the imperial aspirations of earlier eras, while the rhetoric of international peace-keeping goes largely unchallenged, reveals the extent to which Foucault's thesis has become true. While we know there is violence and power at large in the world, it has become invisible, sanitized. We first learnt to split off the violence that was ordinary day-to-day experience several centuries past, vesting it mainly in villains and those who occupy a role of socially sanctioned violence; that is, a policing role. Over centuries, this policing role has been increasingly internalized so that we now police ourselves to be obedient citizens and hardly notice any more the extent to which violence is ingrained in our social ceremonies, our macro-economic systems and our international relations. And we certainly no longer have holy wars – instead, we implement strategies to degrade the weapons-producing capabilities of Third-World tyrannies we had previously armed, effecting only minimal collateral damage in the process. It somehow escapes our notice that we do this using weapons of mass destruction. At the micro-social level too we manage to disavow the violence we do to each other. Although all of the contributors to this text might share this view to some extent, Judi Chamberlin perhaps describes most eloquently the way she finally colluded with the violence done to her experience by the psychiatric system, policing her own extreme emotional states with a vigilance and pathologising gaze as effective as brain-washing.

Although *mental health* is obviously the focus of this text, we have only alluded to it. But in the context of the concluding remarks so far, the reader might glean that in the circumstances described, our view of what constitutes *mental health* goes a long way beyond the absence in an individual of what a psychiatrist would classify as symptoms. Context plays an inescapable part. As Laing encouraged us all those decades ago, we might do well to consider:

> ...the condition of alienation, of being asleep, of being unconscious, of being out of one's mind, ... of ... normal men [who] have killed perhaps 100,000,000 of their fellow men in the last fifty years. (Laing, 1967, pp. 25–30)

> Although one may be inclined to insist that someone whose experience is psychotic appears in some significant way to be 'ill', while the rest of us are not, the most this can really mean is that they are statistically abnormal, for example like a plane no longer flying in formation with the rest of a squadron of planes. Laing urged us not to make the mistake of assuming that society (the rest of the planes still flying 'in formation') is 'on course' and therefore in any particularly superior position (Laing, 1967, pp. 55–76). (Davidson, 1998)

Although our references to Buddhist views may give us away, we will, nonetheless, *not* prescribe any particular view of what mental health is. For now, we feel it is enough to highlight the way in which the concept is so blithely employed, but so rarely defined. What *mental health* actually *is* remains an open question upon which we invite the reader to reflect. Surely, though, the most urgent need of our authors to define for themselves this esoteric phenomenon, and the struggles they have shared with us in the preceding chapters in the pursuit of such a definition, renders their deliberations on the subject and their testimony particularly valid.

Paradoxically, what we have initially taken as our starting point is the diagnosis of *mental illness*, especially in its more severe, psychotic forms. That was the thread that united all the authors, although the patterns of recovery and transcendence they each wove with that thread differed greatly.

Yet this book was, ultimately, about mental health, since that is where the authors all, ultimately, have taken themselves, through their remarkable, and sometimes miraculous, resurrections from the ashes of their experience of what some call madness.

Close Encounters

This book is about experience, and all of the authors have had (often, repeated) encounters with experiences which most people encounter only in dreams. We need to consider carefully not only what might be the messages for the individual authors who have had such experiences, but, also, what might be the messages for the rest of us.

Fifty years ago Aldous Huxley took his first step through *The Doors of Perception* with mescalin, where he saw:

> ...eternity in a flower, infinity in four chair legs and the Absolute in a pair of flannel trousers. Mescalin is the most extraordinary and significant experience available to human beings this side of the Beatific Vision. (Huxley, 1954, p. 27)

W. B. Yeats took a similar trip and was fascinated by a Bovril advertisement on the Thames Embankment. Through doors of altered perception he saw no ordinary advert, but one with gorgeous dragons 'puffing out their breath in front of them in white lines of steam on which white balls were balanced'.

Huxley and Yeats were, of course, by no means the first to try the handle of that door. However, the way that they gained entry was special. Soon, psychopharmacology would attempt to explain how that threshold of perception had been crossed, and in that explanation would lie the paradox of attraction and threat. The theologian Michael Mayne reflected on the history of our 'aspirations' towards contact with the ineffable, aspirations towards the mysteries of planes of consciousness beyond the mundane, and aspirations towards the search to escape the ordinariness of life (Mayne, 1995). Where once such journeys – the spiritual quest – were undertaken through rigorous application, perhaps to the accompaniment of denials of the flesh, stepping through the doors of perception can, now, be a much easier undertaking; perhaps too easy. 'The psychological reorientation after taking drugs can be extremely frightening', Mayne noted 'and, after a period, destructive of the human psyche.' However, the *bad trip* may not simply be a warning for those who seek the easy wisdom of recreational psychedelic drug use. It may be more symbolic, warning everyone of the responsibility that befalls all who step through those doors of perception.

Many of our contributors would define the psychotic journey as an altered state of consciousness that was, for them at least, ultimately spiritual in nature. And for Mayne, the spiritual journey is not one taken lightly. It is no afternoon stroll, but is likely to be a long haul, with many probable detours, obstacles and privations. Indeed, most might at some stage wish that the journey had never been undertaken in the first place. We should take care not to romanticize the distress so evocatively described here. However, those who experience such alterations of consciousness solely as impositions, to be relieved as quickly and efficiently as possible, are by definition retreating from the experience. In contrast with which, many of the authors represented here appear to accept the experience of psychosis. In that acceptance, perhaps, lies the key to their owning and prospering from the experience. In their effort to understand – rather than simply relieve – their distress, one might say that these authors transfigured their experience of ordinary madness into a spiritual undertaking.

Even those authors who did not define their experiences in spiritual terms ultimately emerged from their madness with a new attitude to life and had learned how to see with new eyes. Although we did not select the authors with that criterion in mind, all have described how they found a new commitment to helping others journey through madness. Somehow, as a function of their own emergence, they discovered the value of helping others to emerge into new dawns. Ironically, for people so harshly dealt with by the Fates, all experienced something of what Mayne refers to as a growth in love:

> ...spirituality means growing into the kind of being God has created you to be. It is not simply a matter of widening our consciousness of reality (which drugs may do) but of coming to a more profound and rich aware-ness of things; not an altered consciousness, but a new attitude to life, and a growth in love because you have learned how to see with new eyes. (Mayne, 1995, pp.42–43)

This is a far cry from the pop-spirituality characterizing New Ageism, which differs little from aerobics or any of the 1001 other short-cuts to self-improvement fuelled by ego and destined for the bonfire of the vanities. Having stepped through the special door of perception of the psychotic visitation, our authors have seen the world with very different eyes. Having stepped back through that doorway again into what might be called the consensual reality (Podvoll, 1991) they saw the rest of us not only more clearly, but also more compassionately. Our authors were trans-formed into 'wounded healers' (Barker, 1998).

As far as we are aware, all our authors continue to confront the daily business of being and doing. Although they appear to have made some remarkable discoveries about themselves, their possibilities, and the challenges of living in a curiously uncaring world, they have not 'solved' life or moved into some more esoteric realm of existence. Instead, they have made it their business to draw our attention to what, patently, does not 'work' for those in great psychic distress.

What, then, are the circumstances that best facilitate the sort of attitude to psychotic experience through which it might be seen as epiphany, as spiritual opportunity, as opposed to overwhelming psychic crisis or disaster?

Survivorship, Recovery and Transcendence

If we are not careful, the reader might misinterpret the references to spiritual encounter and growth as suggestions that we should do nothing for someone in distress; that the person should be left to deal with the experience, for it is a stimulus for change. Instead, we believe that there are many things that 'need' to be done, and quite a few others that 'might' be done. The stories published here do, however, highlight one of the great paradoxes of human helping, especially of psychotherapy. Virtually *anything* appears to be of help to someone, but *no one thing* is of help to everyone.

To quote Alan Brownbill, a psychiatric nurse and psychiatric service user, in conversation (on an Internet discussion group for psychiatric nurses) regarding the employment of psychiatric service users:

> I attended a conference recently where a speaker (Jim Read, Mental Health Consultant and Survivor of The Mental Health System) talked about this issue. He asks people: if they had a crisis where they felt overwhelmed by bad feelings or they had lost their ability to function in the world, what they would want? ...the answers tend to be similar no matter who he is asking. They tend to want quiet, comfort, nice surroundings, being close to family and friends, clear information, someone they can trust, somewhere where it is OK to scream, practical help, and sometimes medication if necessary. I think I am right in remembering him saying that nobody has ever said that they would like an acute admission ward in a psychiatric unit. And yet this is so often what is offered. Of course it would be wonderful if an acute admission ward provided the above but I don't know of any that do. ...So much of mental health care provision is imposed from the supposed well to the supposed sick. It is time we took our customers seriously. If we were running a shop with as much arrogance regarding knowing what people want, we would be out of business in no time at all. (Brownbill, 1997)

To paraphrase Brownbill, who seems to have captured the thrust of most of our authors rather well, people don't want therapy, or any type of treatment for that matter, *done to them* (at least not in the first instance); they want validation, support and someone to be a kind of fellow-pilgrim (Read and Reynolds, 1996). Beyond that, they want a life, with support if necessary, to access work, education and so on. Above all, people in states of mental illness want choice, respect and belonging (Rogers et al., 1993).

Community, Relationships and Advocacy

In his classic text, *Escape from Loneliness* (1962), Paul Tournier considered at some length the challenge of loneliness, and its relationship to the erosion of fellowship or *community*. As a physician, he was particularly interested in how people brought to his surgery their loneliness and the problems it generated. He acknowledged that he had written the book 'because the emotional loneliness of modern man had deeply impressed me'. He quoted a colleague who saw the doctor's task as 'nothing less than a complete change of attitude in the patient' (Tournier, 1962, p. 29). It is notable that Tournier's book first appeared fifty years ago, and at the time he saw the problem of emotional loneliness as essentially European in character. Perhaps its shadow has now spread more widely, or perhaps Tournier was being unduly European in claiming the problem for his own peoples. Certainly the authors represented here, from the USA, UK and Australia, all describe a sense of alone-ness with their psychic distress. Indeed, their alienation and isolation were often confirmed best by the feckless efforts of psychiatric professionals to produce the 'change of attitude' referred to by Tournier. What they needed, when at the nadir of the psychotic journey, was fellowship, not treatment: someone to join *with* them, not to act *upon* them. Tournier saw a fine example of such conjoint caring in Hippocrates:

> When men saw wood, one man pulls toward himself, while the other pushes; yet they actually do the same thing. Opposite movements are necessary if the saw is to cut through the wood. If the two men tried to use their strength without harmonising their activities, chaos would result. (Tournier, 1962, p. 186)

There are too many references to such organized chaos in the narratives published here. Too many of the authors were repeatedly denied the kind of relationship that might both validate their distress, and begin to cut through the ties that bound them. Perhaps many such misunderstandings about what 'needs to be done', in caring about and relating to people in great mental distress, involve the illusion of duality. Professional helpers assume that the 'patient' and all her/his experiences are alien; they represent something that can be related to only from a great distance. No wonder that the 'patient' feels alienated, isolated or cut adrift. As we noted in our introduction, the basis of such dualism is fear: professionals fear the 'other' that the patient represents. And fear is not an emotion that can be dealt with effectively without liberal challenges by trust, love and faith. Perhaps the authors here emerged from their psychotic nightmares because they found their own capacities to trust and love themselves. In the process they found, perhaps, the faith that is the root of all effective psychiatric rescues. Perhaps mental health professionals do not need new psychological tools, so much as old human ones: the capacities to display trust, to express love and to have faith – faith in themselves, faith in their own potential for human growth and development and also faith that the person they are helping will emerge, relatively unscathed, from their journey.

References

Barker P (1998) Creativity and psychic distress in writers artists and scientists. Journal of Psychiatric and Mental Health Nursing 5(2): 109–118.

Brownbill A (1997) Subject: Re: Users of the Service; Date: Tue, 17 Jun 1997 08:12:51 +0000; from: A.I.Brownbill@herts.ac.uk (Alan Brownbill); sender: psychiatric-nursing-request@mailbase.ac.uk

Davidson B (1998) The role of the psychiatric nurse. In Barker P, Davidson B (Eds) Psychiatric Nursing: Ethical Strife. Arnold, London, ch.5, pp 57–65.

Huxley A (1954) The Doors of Perception. London: Chatto & Windus.

Laing RD (1967) The Politics of Experience. Harmondsworth: Penguin.

Mayne M (1995) This Sunrise of Wonder: Letters for the Journey. London: Fount-HarperCollins.

Podvoll E (1991) The Seduction of Madness: A Compassionate Approach to Recovery from Psychosis at Home. London: Century.

Read J, Reynolds J (1996) Speaking our Minds: An Anthology of Personal Experiences of Mental Distress and its Consequences. London: Macmillan, and Milton Keynes: Open University Press.

Rogers, Pilgrim and Lacey (1993) Experiencing Psychiatry – Users Views of Services. London: Macmillan & MIND.

Tournier P (1962) Escape from Loneliness. London: SCM Press.

Index

Main Line Emergency
610-642-1160
Eliz +